# Competition in the Marketplace: Health Care in the 1980s

**Monographs in Health Care Administration**
*Series editor,* **Samuel Levy, Ph.D.,** University of Iowa

Volume 1:
**Competition in the Marketplace: Health Care in the 1980s**
*Edited by James Gay and Barbara Sax Jacobs*

# Competition in the Marketplace: Health Care in the 1980s

*Edited by*

**James R. Gay, M.D.**
**Barbara J. Sax Jacobs, J.D.**

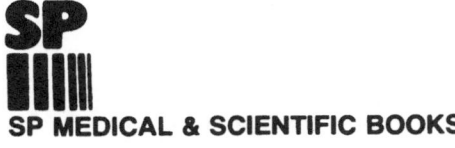

**SP MEDICAL & SCIENTIFIC BOOKS**

New York

SPECTRUM PUBLICATIONS, INC.
175-20 Wexford Terrace, Jamaica, N.Y. 11432


Gay, James, ed.
  Competition in the marketplace.

  Jamaica, NY: Spectrum Publications
Library of Congress Catalog Card No.: 81-85561
ISBN  978-94-011-7395-7          ISBN  978-94-011-7393-3  (eBook)
DOI 10.1007/978-94-011-7393-3

# The Frank Norfleet Forum
# for the Advancement of Health

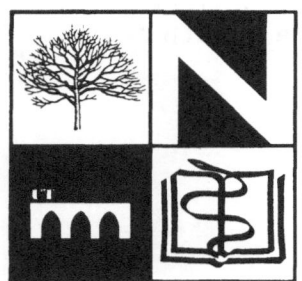

## THE UNIVERSITY OF TENNESSEE
## CENTER FOR THE HEALTH SCIENCES

James R. Gay, M.D., Editor
Associate Vice President for Health Affairs
The University of Tennessee


Barbara J. Sax Jacobs, J.D., Editor
Research Associate (Administration)
Office of the Vice Chancellor for
Academic Affairs
The University of Tennessee
Center for the Health Sciences


Cynthia Brock Kent, Administrative Secretary
Office of Special Programs
The University of Tennessee
Center for the Health Sciences


Kay W. Cowell, Supervisor
Word Processing Center
The University of Tennessee
Center for the Health Sciences

# ACKNOWLEDGEMENTS

The Norfleet Forum is the product of many dedicated persons. Dozens of The University of Tennessee staff members willingly performed the tasks needed for the production of the first Norfleet Forum. The Chancellor, the Director and the Trustees are very grateful for their unselfish efforts.

Donations to the Forum are continuing from persons other than the original donor. Thus, the continuity of active participation of the University of Tennessee in national health policymaking is assured. The University appreciates their thoughtful concern.

The Director wishes to thank Barbara J. Sax Jacobs, who assumed major responsibility for editing the proceedings, with the assistance of Cynthia Brock Kent, Kay W. Cowell and Melinda Thomas, who assisted in preparation of the manuscript. Their expertise and devotion were critical elements in the process of publishing these proceedings.

The former Chancellor, T. Albert Farmer, Jr., M.D.; the current Chancellor, James C. Hunt, M.D.; Bland W. Cannon, Advisor to the Chancellor; C. E. "Mickey" Bilbrey, Vice Chancellor for Development; John K. Fockler, Executive Director of Memphis-Plough Community Foundation; and each of the Trustees named in the proceedings assumed a full share of the responsibilities. The Director for the Forum thanks each of them for their continuing interest and support.


The Editors express their appreciation to Maurice Ancharoff of Spectrum Publications, Incorporated, for his interest, cooperation and patience.

# Contributors

Robert D. Burnett, M.D.
Sunnyvale, California


Robert A. Derzon
Lewin and Associates, Inc.
Washington, D.C.


The Honorable David F. Durenberger
United States Senate
Washington, D.C.


Merlin K. DuVal, M.D.
National Center for Health Education
San Francisco, California


Paul M. Ellwood, M.D.
InterStudy
Excelsior, Minnesota


Alain C. Enthoven, Ph.D.
Stanford University
Stanford, California


W. T. Johnston
Department of Human Services
Project Health Division
Portland, Oregon


Walter McClure, Ph.D.
InterStudy
Excelsior, Minnesota


Glenn Nelson, M.D.
St. Louis Park Medical Center
Minneapolis, Minnesota


Tom E. Nesbitt, Jr., M.D.
American Medical Association
Nashville, Tennessee

Carl J. Schramm, Ph.D., J.D.
The Johns Hopkins Medical Institutions
Baltimore, Maryland


John A. Shively, M.D.
The University of Tennessee
Center for the Health Sciences
Memphis, Tennessee


Henry E. Simmons, M.D.
Peat, Marwick, Mitchell & Co.
Washington, D.C.


Frank A. Sloan, Ph.D.
Vanderbilt University
Nashville, Tennessee


Jesse H. Turner, Sr.
Shelby County Commissioner
Memphis, Tennessee

# FOREWORD

The first Frank M. Norfleet Forum for the Advancement of Health was convened December 1-3, 1980 at The University of Tennessee Center for the Health Sciences, Memphis.

It is an annual invitational forum created to focus on the improvement of health status in the community, state, nation and world through effective health policies and organizations.

As issues of health care become more complex, the Norfleet Forum is expected to serve as a vehicle for discussion and dissemination of information needed by policymakers and administrators in selecting intricate solutions to health care problems.

It is administered by a five member board of trustees, including two members from the Memphis-Plough Community Foundation's board of governors and three representatives of The University of Tennessee Center for the Health Sciences.

This Forum is made possible by the generous gift of Dunbar Abston, Sr., and is named in honor of his adopted stepson, Frank M. Norfleet. Mr. Abston enjoys a business career associated with Parts Industries Corporation of Memphis, one of the largest automotive parts supply and equipment distributors in the nation. Frank M. Norfleet is interested in the welfare of the Memphis community and is particularly active in health affairs. He served as the first chairman of the Mid-South Medical Center Council and as chairman of The University of Tennessee Center for the Health Sciences Chancellor's Round Table. Mr. Norfleet is President and chief executive officer of Parts Industries Corporation of Memphis and is a member of the board of directors of several national business organizations.

The competitive model for containing costs and assuring high quality of medical care continues to occupy the attention of economists, strategic planners and policymakers. The principle advocates of competition and prepaid multi-specialty group practice systems report their ideas in these proceedings. It is apparent from hearing and reading what they are saying that competition is progressing far beyond being just a theoretical concept. In many metropolitan areas of the west, southwest, central and northeast sections of the nation, the number of prepaid group practices are expanding, and they are competing with each other for a share of the medical care business. The proposition that competition can control costs and at the same time provide excellent medical care is being tested in the marketplace.

James R. Gay, M.D.
Director, Norfleet Forum

# TABLE OF CONTENTS

# INTRODUCTION
# T. Albert Farmer, Jr.

The Norfleet Forum has been made possible by two men. The endowment that supports this annual invitational forum on health policy issues was made through the great generosity of Mr. Dunbar Abston. There is no one in the Memphis community who could more appropriately be chosen to have the Forum bear his name than Frank M. Norfleet. He is a man widely respected in the community by men and by women, by the affluent and by the poor, by the white and by the black, all of whom have directly or indirectly benefited from his continuing sense of civic responsibility.

This annual forum on selected issues related to health care will not only serve as a platform to debate, discuss and evaluate the timely issues in health care, but will provide a unique opportunity for The University of Tennessee to assemble a special group of national experts, key involved individuals and dedicated local citizens concerned with a specific health policy issue.

The timeliness of this year's topic, "Health Care in the 1980s: Competition in the Marketplace," is evident because to whatever extent and in whatever manner it is implemented, the competition approach to the provision of health care services in the United States must be addressed and must be addressed now.

Americans face a predicament in the present health care system, and this is the predicament of uncontrollable costs in a system that still has inadequate access for millions of individuals. The passive third-party role in fee-for-service physician reimbursement and hospital cost reimbursement not only provides no rewards for economy but has eliminated the price controlling effect of the usual marketplace concept that Americans understand. In spite of these rapidly increasing costs, there are more than 20 million Americans with no insurance and another 20 to 30 million with inadequate insurance coverage.

Attention must be focused to the real options available. Continued rhetoric concerning unrealistic options will not solve the problems. Voluntary efforts that have been made in recent years are laudable but cannot solve the basic problems. A totally free market that is non-regulated is completely untenable and would cause disastrous preferred risk selection problems. A totally government financed and operated system is not only unacceptable to the American people but cannot be implemented in our free enterprise society.

There are only two options, and those are regulation by increasing rate control or regulations that encourage competition and restore workable marketplace principles.

During the Forum, the advantages of the competition approach, the secondary benefits from such an approach that provide incentives to cut costs, and the possible mechanisms for how this might be accomplished will be discussed.

As an individual who believes strongly in the long-range value of the competitive approach over the rate regulatory approach, I want to take this opportunity to encourage the distinguished speakers and participants to plan these changes in a way that prevents disasters that could occur if certain issues are not addressed. As I have spoken to civic clubs and written articles, even in the Memphis newspapers, encouraging marketplace initiatives, I worry that we will not properly address the danger of shifting our focus from quality to economics. I further worry that we may reverse the trend away from a two-class care system unless good minimal acceptable standards are imposed. I further worry that we may see great disruptions as individuals try to understand and choose if we do not give them the proper assistance to do so.

I have a particular bias and a particular concern for the future of our academic health science centers because of the ease with which government can regulate such institutions.

As patient referrals are shifted to advanced secondary level hospitals or within developing discrete hospital networks, what will happen to university hospitals? Where will the development of new procedures and technology occur if university hospitals are lost? How will high cost, low volume, specialized services, such as the 50 percent of burn units and 44 percent of transplant units located in university hospitals, be provided? Who will render the care to the indigent, a major responsibility of university hospitals?

Even beyond these important questions, a more vital question that must be addressed is how graduate medical education and allied health education costs that are now primarily financed by university hospitals from the patient care dollar will be financed? With the danger of these kinds of costs making university hospitals non-competitive, the quality of care will be in serious jeopardy because in the long run it is people who determine quality. If the approximately 215,000 health professionals currently in training in university hospitals are not well-trained, Americans cannot have a quality care system.

These are vital issues that must be addressed and resolved because a competitive approach has long-range advantages over a regulatory system in both controlling costs and improving access to care.

# Competition in the Marketplace: Health Care in the 1980s

# I
# THE POLITICS OF HEALTH
## David F. Durenberger

I want to congratulate everyone who is taking part in the conference. I suspect that a lot of the people are where I was a few
years ago when I started to get involved in health care issues.
I did not know what the answers were, but I knew something had to
be done about our country's health care delivery system.

I listened to some of the same people speaking at this conference
--Alain Enthoven, Paul Ellwood, Walt McClure and Glen Nelson --
saw what was happening in my home state of Minnesota, and came to
the conclusion that competition and consumer choice were the answers. I hope that at the end of this Forum the participants come
to the same conclusion. But, the important thing is that everyone look for new ideas and new ways to deliver necessary health
care services.

This is the key. Because out of the search for better answers,
new and better ways of delivering health care and other social
services will be found.

Many at the Forum are looking for new answers because of what has
been happening in this country, not only in the last decade, but
in the last few months.

Politicians, both those in office and those trying to get there,
have made a lot of promises this year. This was going to be the
year of the balanced budget. We know now, some of us knew ten
months ago, that we are not going to have a balanced budget.
In fact, recently Congress proposed a $633 billion budget with a
deficit of at least $27 billion, or if everything goes wrong, a
deficit that could be as high as $75 billion for fiscal 1981.

Yet, the American people are still getting promises:

$39 billion in tax cuts;

A five to eleven percent increase in defense spending;

A reduction in inflation and the interest rates on borrowed money; and

New jobs added to the economy and the unemployed put back to work.

We are here at this Forum to discuss how access to health care can be improved in a country whose health care bill last year reached $212 billion making it the nation's third largest industry. Health care costs were an average of $943 per person, the highest in the world. Yet, despite that huge investment, the United States is not yet among the top ten countries in the world in such measures as life expectancy and infant mortality.

How are we going to make good on all these promises and improve access to affordable public services, including health care? The answer is in our history, the message of the last few national elections, and the reasons for this Forum--the role of government must be changed.

We are several years into the kind of fundamental change that has taken place about every 100 years in this country. Going back to the Boston Tea Party, not only was a lot of tea kicked into the Boston Harbor, but King George was kicked out of this country. Americans said, "Look, we came to this country for a reason. We not only want the freedom to grow our tobacco, we want the freedom to sell it on our terms wherever we can get the best price."

That tea party helped give birth to a nation of people who wanted to let individuality and free enterprise flourish, and who did not want a lot of government because they had had enough government from King George.

That nation of individuality did flourish. But after a hundred years, the robber barons were exploiting its human resources for cheap labor and its natural resources for material, and were destroying its communities in the process. The rights and opportunities of the majority were being sacrificed to the success of a few--the few who owned the railroads, the steel mills, the oil companies and the other major industries.

The interests of the public and of the community against the dominant power of private interests needed to be asserted. So, Americans turned to government, especially to the national government, for leadership. Decisions were made increasingly through the forum of politics and carried out increasingly through the process of bureaucracy.

Teddy Roosevelt, a Republican by the way, articulated the idea of a strong national government operating in the interests of the common people in his concept of a "New Nationalism." After the New Nationalism came Woodrow Wilson's "New Freedom," Franklin Roose-

velt's "New Deal," Harry Truman's "Fair Deal," and John Kennedy's
"New Frontier." Through all these programs, the national government used its vast resources to gain more and more control over
services that were once delivered privately or by local governments. Federal aid to education, urban redevelopment, the use and
protection of land, air and water, human and social services, and
hundreds of other programs were all gathered under the national
thumb, not only through control of the dollar in Washington, but
through a multitude of rules and regulations.

Two years ago Proposition 13 occurred which was nothing more than
a group of Californians telling government, "You've done too much
for us. Leave us alone for awhile."

That was the same message some politicians heard in the 1976 national election--but Jimmy Carter never got the word. At the
least when people voted for Ronald Reagan and all the minority party candidates throughout the country, they were saying, "I want to
change the role of government. From now on, I want more of a say
in my own future."

That is the same thing they said to Jimmy Carter when he was cam-
paigning by telling people all the right things. He was going to
make government smaller; he was going to balance the budget; and he
was going to cut taxes and the bureaucracy. But, Jimmy Carter made
one fundamental mistake and made it right in the beginning. He
came to Washington with armloads of big blue books telling him all
there was to know about the national government. And he never got
out of the books. He never stopped trying to run the government.
He never did get the real message of his own election or of Proposition 13. So, in 1980 this country threw out an elected incum-
bent President for the first time since 1932.

Now, everyone has to respond to the 1980 election by changing the
role of government. A variety of solutions have been offered.
One cure says that there is nothing wrong with the system, it is
simply a problem of the people who are running it. Another cure
says the people are okay, but the system has to be reformed. And
the more radical approach suggests that spending and taxing limita-
tions, preferably through constitutional amendment, will best improve government.

Frankly, I think the last one is necessary, but I also think that
is the easy part. The 97th Congress will reform the way and the
amount of money we collect and spend. We will provide incentives
to enourage Americans to save and invest more of their dollars instead of spending them as soon as they are earned. We will accomplish all those things, but it will not be enough. It will not
balance the budget, or reduce inflation, or lower interest rates.
Only radical change in the way this nation provides access to quality and affordable public services for its citizens can do that,
and that means change the role of government in the delivery of
public services.

I will speak briefly about how an institution as big as the national government can be changed. There are two alternative ways

to correct an institution's failing behavior. People can talk out
the problems, or they can walk away. The former is called "voice;"
the latter is "exit."

There are many opportunities for voice--everything from local
planning commissions to forums such as this one. As more and more
activities and more and more people migrate into the public sector,
they become stakeholders who decide to stay and talk it out rather
than exiting.

The whole system actually would work better if it would realize
that exit is needed to make voice more effective. In other words,
protest against the system makes protest within the system more
powerful. Each approach makes the system more accountable.

The system developed to provide public services relies too much
on voice and not enough on exit. Americans cannot exit because
there is no place to go; there are too few alternative delivery
systems. So, they stay and talk it out and the result has been
more government regulation, more subsidization, greater budget de-
ficits and reduced quality of services.

In health care and other services more opportunity for exit must
be provided. Give the consumers more choices to exit from one
plan and move to another. Let the users determine which delivery
systems will survive.

That is the choice to make when we look at the two schools of
thought that have emerged on the crisis of health care. The lines
are drawn between those on one side who favor more government involvement through subsidization and regulation, and those on the
other side, including me, who believe that our health care needs
will best be met by instilling the marketplace concepts of competition and consumer choice. These two schools represent the difference between saying the system is basically sound, it just
needs some fine tuning; and saying there is a better way to deliver
the service.

The Carter Administration, its Republican predecessors and others
have opted for the regulatory approach. Certificate-of-need, rate
review programs and recent attempts at cost containment are prime
examples of government attempts to control health care costs through
regulation aimed at hospitals. There is no question that government regulations themselves have done little to address the basic
problems in the delivery system. Instead, they have actually con-
tributed to health inflation.

A major problem with the regulatory approach is that it overlooks
the fact that most health care services do not have cost sensitive
consumers because health care consumers do not choose a service,
they choose a doctor. Then the doctor determines the hospital to
which the patient will be admitted, the tests to be ordered, and
the treatments to be prescribed. There is little economic reward
for the physician who practices a cost-effective style of medicine; who keeps patients healthy and out of the hospital; or who
uses the most cost-effective hospital when such care is needed.

In fact, the reverse is usually true. Why shouldn't the physician use the most luxurious and expensive hospital in town? It is nicer for the physician and the patient, and the patient's insurance pays for it anyway.

That point is missed by the regulators. The regulators see all the problems as being the same and, consequently, they cannot distinguish among the solutions. The regulatory approach, by necessity, is aimed at correcting a specific problem in a general setting. A problem in one city may not exist in another, or a shortcoming of one hospital may be a strength of another. Yet, both groups are forced to comply with the same regulations.

Regulation in many ways is an outgrowth of government subsidization of health care. Since the 1940s and 50s, government has been the driving force behind the effort to fill hospital beds. The national government has subsidized health care through Medicare, incentives to train new medical personnel, hospital construction, tax subsidies for health coverage and a host of other programs.

This massive subsidization has taken cost control out of the marketplace. In this system of national subsidization of health care, regulation is the only way to keep down costs.

The answer is to change the way health care is delivered by changing the way health care is choosen and paid for.

Meaningful competition may just be the last defense against regulation and subsidization. The kinds of activity taking place in Minneapolis/St. Paul and elsewhere need to be explored and expanded in other areas of the country. The legislation I introduced last year, the Health Incentives Reform Act, is designed to do just that.

The bill was called the Health Incentives Reform Act because that is exactly what I hope it will accomplish: reform the incentives which affect the delivery of health care.

The bill proposes to increase competition with several key provisions. First, it amends the Internal Revenue Code to provide that unless employers of over 100 persons who pay for employee health care offer at least three health plans, each from a different carrier, their employees will pay income tax on the employer's health care contribution. By choosing the employers of more than 100 persons, about one-half of the total work force will be covered. More important, I believe that the bill provides the necessary starting point and that its ripples will spread throughout the entire population.

Second, the bill provides that to keep contributions tax-free, employers must contribute equally to each plan. This guarantees that the employee's choice of health plans is not influenced by the amount of the employer contribution.

Third, it reduces the government subsidization of very expensive plans by limiting the tax deductability of the employer contribu-

tion.  The limit proposed in 1980 was $125 per month for a family
of four, but the actual figure is not as important as the concept.
The important thing is to limit tax subsidization to a level consistent with the public well-being.  If more expensive plans are
desired, that is fine, but they should be financed through wages,
not tax subsidies.

Fourth, the bill mandates catastrophic coverage.  Every person has
the right to be protected from the effects of a catastrophic illness or accident that threatens not only his health but his financial security.  The bill requires all plans to meet certain minimum standards to qualify for tax exemption.  Included in these standards are continuity of coverage after death, divorce or termina-
tion of employment, and the right to purchase dependent coverage
and catastrophic coverage.

Fifth, the bill requires all health plans to limit consumer out-
of-pocket expenses for basic benefits to a maximum annual amount.

It is critical to the success of competitive health care to involve
employers in the selection of plans.  That belief is substantiated
by a recent Lou Harris survey that said most members of health maintenance organizations (HMO) are enrolled in HMOs through their
own employer or union or through the employer or union of a family
member.

That poll also helps debunk the idea that an alternative health
care system will deliver cut-rate services.  Seventy-five percent
of the HMO members surveyed said they "certainly will" renew their
membership and another 17 percent said they "probably will" renew.

Competition and consumer choice will change the way health care
is delivered because it will put the decision-making process in
the hands of the community--the individual citizen, the employer
and business, and the local marketplace.  Competition and consumer
choice encourage local, voluntary, community based cost control
mechanisms.  They also provide the alternative vehicles on which
to piggyback subsidized care for the poor as access is expanded
to everyone in the country.

I fully expect these pro-competitive provisions to receive serious
consideration in 1981 and to be passed by the 97th Congress.  But,
whether they are passed next year or two or three years from now,
there is no doubt in my mind that competition and consumer choice
are the wave of the future.

Competition and consumer choice will force us to look at the entire
field of health care in a new light, just as we finally saw the
light and governed government out of energy pricing in this country.  We have to get the government out of the business of making
price decisions through the regulatory process or subsidization.

The role of government in health manpower must be questioned.  Can
the marketplace determine the number and special skills of doctors
needed?  As the definition of the word "hospital" changes, the role
of government in subsidizing the construction of hospitals must

be questioned. Could that job be better left to communities and trustees who are reacting to need rather than to artificial costs?

Government, of course, will not abdicate its role in meeting the need of everyone in this nation for access to affordable health care. But, government's role will be changed to that of a policy-maker. The users of health care services, consumers and communities, will make the decision on how to implement the policies set by government.

In a competitive environment, hospitals, for example, must be led by their trustees and managers to look beyond the four walls of their building. The successful hospital will be the one in which the managers have ceased to define their hospital by the physical facility, but define it by the service it offers. Hospitals in a competitive society must become less of a building and more of a health and sickness corporation. For too long, hospitals have concentrated only on acute care with the need to fill as many beds as possible. That approach is no longer viable in a cost conscious environment. Hospitals must go beyond that to offer a range of health and sickness services, including mental health, family counseling, chemical dependency programs, and outpatient and long-term care.

As to long-term care, hospitals are going to be challenged to plan not only in their own best interest--filling their beds--but in the interest of the community. Recently, my health task force held a meeting in Minnesota and focused mostly on the issue of long-term care. The areas they emphasized in considering legislative solutions to the problems of long-term care are flexibility, local control, and initiative. I could not agree more.

We have to look at long-term care in a new light. The Senate and House conferees working out differences in the fiscal 1981 budget reconciliation agreed to a Senate provision to reimburse hospitals providing long-term care at the skilled nursing or intermediate care facility rate.

The so-called swing bed provision applies to small rural hospitals and to patients determined to need non-acute services rather than hospital care, but where no long-term care beds are available. Savings are estimated at $101 million in fiscal 1981.

That may be one approach, but it is not the only answer. We have to resolve the problems that force some Medicare beneficiaries into hospitals for three days before they can be reimbursed for nursing home care. We have to find answers that do not just fill beds, but meet patients' needs.

There is no question that more efficient ways to provide care must be developed. Home care should be able to compete with hospitals, nursing homes and other facilities. The issue is whether such care is less costly. If it just skims patients, there is no clear advantage. That is, if hospitals can care for those who need this limited care just as cheaply, then they might be encouraged to do so. Medicare cost allocations, however, may preclude this. That

is why we should let the users make the choice, not the policy-
makers.

Other changes will certainly be brought about by health care plan-
ning--letting the community decide.   Good health care planning
will establish broad rules for fair competition and will help us
look into the future so that those providing health care can respond adequately to the needs of individuals.

Planning is not an effort to satisfy public wants, but rather to
establish needs.   Planning under competition can change its role
to that of a consumer advocate helping consumers get the best
values in medical care.

Competition in health care changes the incentives we now have.
The incentives in a competitive environment are to keep people
healthy, whether it is through an HMO that stresses preventive
care or an employer-based wellness program.

Wellness is the key.  Right now, the only time a secretary receives
flowers is during National Secretary Week or when she is in the
hospital.  A wellness program rewards the people who take care of
themselves, the people who stay healthy.   Instead of sick days,
there should be health days.  While consoling those who are ill,
there should be rewards for those who are healthy.

Employers, through a wellness program, can do a great deal to promote good health.  And, a wellness program is something that can
be started right now, without waiting for changes in government
regulations or subsidization.

The national government's first priority as we move to a competitive environment must be to control inflation.   Unless inflation
is under control, everything else is impossible to accomplish because inflation robs individuals and local communities of the economic freedom of choice that is essential to competition.

In the same vein, the second priority of the national government
must be to change the income security programs, from welfare to
social security.  These programs must become more flexible and give
consumers the right to make decisions on the services they use.
What good is consumer choice without the financial resources necessary to exercise that choice?  Whether we talk about changing
government's role by introducing the "exit" choice into health care,
education or transportation, we must also solve these two major
societal problems.

Frankly, there is an element of risk in competition.  No one, including the most ardent advocates of competition, know exactly what
it will bring.  No one can predict with complete accuracy the outcome of national policy decisions.  But, we have found the error
in the once held belief that nothing is good unless it comes from
the bureaucracy.  That is a dead-end road.

In the 97th Congress I hope to be not only the chairman of the Finance Subcommittee on Health, but the chairman of the Intergovern-

mental Relations Subcommittee of Governmental Affairs.  One of my
subcommittees will deal with actual health care service, the other
will deal with the way we go about making decisions.  Our task in
the subcommittees will be to meet the challenge of the Reagan pres-
idency:  "America...A New Beginning."

Meeting that challenge begins with an examination of federalism
in America.  In the Nixon years, we heard about a new federalism.
It meant General Revenue Sharing and block grants instead of categorical grants.  It meant shifting power from national to state
government by shifting federal taxes to state spenders.

But, I think the origins of American constitutional history are
misconstrued if they are conceived to be about monolithic struc-
tures--national and state governments.  The key to federalism is
not just shifting tax dollars as was done during the Nixon years.
Rather, the historic key to federalism is separation and division
--separation of power and division of authority.  That means competition, diversity and individuality.  There never was a question
about whether there would be states, only whether there would be
a national government.

I do not have all the answers, but that is not my job.  My job is
to take good ideas and convert them into good legislation.  It is
not going to be easy.  But, if we fail to make our health delivery
system more cost-effective, we will sacrifice quality or accessi-
bility or both.  If we do not take the lead in changing our system,
then we will be the first ones to feel the effects of our failure.

I am confident that we will succeed because I have seen the beginning of that success in Minnesota.  I am confident that the 1980s
will mark the beginning of a new era of more affordable and more
accessible public services, starting with health care.  That must
be our goal.

# II
# COMPETITION IN THE MARKETPLACE: HEALTH CARE IN THE 1980s
## Alain C. Enthoven

I hope the ideas, concepts and experiences discussed at the Nor-fleet Forum will provide a basis on which a health care system to better serve the citizens of Tennessee can be built.

There is no need to belabor the fact that the cost of health care in this country has become a very serious problem. Nationally, health care spending, which was about $43 billion in 1965, reached $245 billion in 1980, going from 6.2 to 9.5 percent of the gross national product. Net of general inflation this meant a doubling in real per capita spending on health care services. During the same period, health care spending by federal, state and local gov-ernments went from $11 billion to $100 billion. Medicare costs alone doubled every four years in the 1970s, going from $9 billion in 1972 to $18 billion in 1976.

President-elect Reagan promised to cut taxes and increase defense spending. It is important to understand that the proposed tax cuts and defense spending increases are responses to fundamental problems and not mere expressions of conservative policy pref-erences. Tax cuts are needed to restore incentives to work, to save, and to make productive investments in order to reverse the decline in productivity in the economy. Defense spending increases are needed to reverse the relative decline in American military power. It seems inevitable that the Reagan administration will have to move forcefully to slow the growth in health care spending to accomplish these goals because this growth adds to inflationary pressures and weakens the competitive position of American indus-try.

Why are health care costs increasing? Many factors are involved. For example, insurance coverage, especially for the aged and the poor, has increased, and there has been a tremendous growth in med-ical technology. One important observation about the increase in spending is that it is not all bad. A lot of it is good, and Amer-

11

cans would not reverse it if they could. However, it is also true that there is a lot of waste, that is, increased spending yielding no discernible improvement in health status. The reason for this is a financing system in which most insured consumers are not cost conscious and in which providers of care are rewarded for cost-increasing behavior. Under the insured fee-for-service system, physicians receive more revenue for providing more costly services whether or not more does the patient any good. For example, a gastroenterologist is also an endoscopist. If a patient comes to him complaining of diarrhea, he can do a colonoscopy, and be reimbursed $400.00 by a third-party payor. On the other hand, if he just talks to the patient to find out what is bothering him and causing the problem, he will receive $40.00. This kind of incentive must affect the way a physician practices.

Similarly, under cost reimbursement, hospitals receive more revenue for generating more costs. There is no reward for being economical. A system has been created for which there are many cost-increasing incentives, but no rewards for economy. Inflation is the predictable result.

During the past decade, the main direction of public policy was to place controls on prices, capacity and utilization of services. This policy resulted in increased bureaucratic involvement in the details of the delivery of health care services, but introduced no force for economy or consumer satisfaction. This regulatory approach, as indicated by the following review, has been an economic and political failure. The Carter administration, unfortunately, devoted practically all of its legislative energies in the health care field to its hospital cost containment proposal—the "9 percent solution." When the proposal came down to the wire in the House of Representatives, it had become little more than symbolic politics, as most hospitals were exempted by one of the provisions added to obtain approval of the bill. In addition, if the bill had passed, the system's incentives would have been perverse because its price control mechanism rewarded the fat and punished the lean. To illustrate, picture two hospitals, one running lean at a rate of $1 million a year, and the other doing the same job for $2 million a year. Applying the 9 percent solution for cost containment, the hospital doing the job for $2 million would receive a $180,000 increase, while the economical hospital would only receive a $90,000 increase.

The Nixon administration's economic stabilization program included such controls, and prospective studies showed that they failed to induce any economy in resource use. One reason for this failure was that price controls very quickly became a cost reimbursement system. Hospital personnel went to the price control authorities complaining that because of rising costs, the hospital would go broke if an extra increase was not allowed. Predictably, the authorities allowed that cost increase to be passed on to the patient.

In the mid-1960s, a certificate-of-need program was enacted in New York state. By 1974, about half the states in this country had such laws. At that point two things happened. One, a number of

health services researchers began to examine whether or not certificate-of-need programs were beneficial.  Second, Congress, without waiting for the results of these studies, passed a law mandat-
ing that every state have a certificate-of-need law by 1980.  Unfortunately, the studies showed that certificate-of-need laws were
ineffective because they (1) blocked innovation, (2) did not shut
down the inefficient producer of services, and (3) provided incentives to keep unneeded capacity open.  In addition, they provided
politicians with an opportunity to gain special interest voter support if the politicians overturned unpopular local certificate-of-
need decisions.

In 1972, Congress, in voluminous amendments to the Social Security
law, enacted the Professional Standards Review Organization program (PSRO).  PSRO established independent bodies of physicians
across the country who would contract with the Department of
Health, Education, and Welfare to review Medicare and Medicaid utilization with the purpose of controlling the costs of these programs.  In the last year, studies have compared geographical areas
with PSROs, with areas that were supposed to have them but did not.
The areas were statistically controlled for relevant variables.
Of the two leading studies, one found that PSROs did not save
enough money to pay for themselves, and the other found that PSROs
just barely saved enough money to cover costs.  Thus, neither study
showed a significant or substantial cost-reducing effect.

There have also been proposals to control physicians' fees.  In
fact, the Nixon administration's Economic Stabilization Program
did so.  The experience under the Economic Stabilization Program
showed that there are many ways for physicians to bypass controls,
for example, by increasing utilization or by unbundling, that is,
billing what was previously billed as one service as two or three
different services.  As  a result, while price controls held down
the growth in fees to less than the inflation rate, the increase
in utilization fully offset the controls and protected the real
incomes of physicians.  In my opinion, controls on physicians' fees
are a particularly unproductive way of controlling health care
costs.  The regulatory approach costs hundreds of millions of dollars, politicizes the industry, focuses attention on beating rules
rather than providing better care at less cost, and does not
reach the fundamental problems of the system.

Before examining non-governmental strategies for cost control, it
is important to note that compared to the costly standard of care
that predominates in many parts of this country, it is possible
to cut costs through organized systems of care without cutting the
quality of care.  One of the main ways is to match resources used
to the needs of the population served.  Victor Fuchs, at Stanford
University, conducted an interesting study on the utilization and
costs of surgery in different parts of the country.  He found that
if you have twice the surgeons per capita in one area as in
another, there will be roughly double the fees and 30 percent
more surgery per capita.  Thus, to organize an economical system
for the delivery of surgical services, an appropriate number of
surgeons is needed such that they will be kept busy and proficient,
and at the same time be able to make a good living while charging
a low fee per case.  This principle of matching resources to needs

can be applied to all types of health care resources, including hospital bed utilization.

Another way to cut costs but not quality is through appropriate regional distribution or concentration of specialized services. A few years ago, a doctoral student at Stanford studied the economics of open heart surgery in California by looking at (1) the cost per case for hospital and surgical teams doing different annual volumes of cases, and (2) the number of cases done at each institution. He found that, on the average, teams that did 50 cases a year cost roughly $20,000 a case, whereas teams doing 500 cases a year, cost $8,000 or $9,000 a case. These are important economies of scale. Furthermore, he found the surgery was performed in 91 hospitals with an average of 160 operations each; 15,000 operations in the state overall. About two-thirds of these 91 hospitals did less than the 150 cases a year recommended by the specialty societies as a minimum for proficiency. In fact, some hospitals did less than 100 or even less than 50 cases a year. He estimated that it would be possible to save $40 million a year in California alone if all open heart surgery were concentrated in 30 centers each doing about 500 cases a year.

A recent article in the New England Journal of Medicine by Hal Luft, John Bunker, and myself examined the relationship between surgical mortality and volume for about a dozen surgical procedures, ranging from the very complex to the very simple. In the case of open heart surgery we found a very pronounced relationship between surgical mortality and the volume of operations done by the hospital. Roughly, at 50 operations a year, the mortality rate was ten or eleven percent. At 200 or 300 operations per year, the mortality rate was perhaps six percent.

These two studies suggest that it would be possible for Californians to have better results, lower surgical mortality, and also lower costs, if there were a rational distribution of heart surgery in the state. This model for economy could be applied to many specialized services, for example, radiation therapy and laboratory services.

A third way to cut costs is to reduce the rate of hospital utilization per capita to an appropriate amount which would be considerably below the present norm. There are a number of prominent organized systems of health care delivery in this country in which hospital days per 1000 people per year are, on the average, roughly 40 percent less than the national average for a similar group of patients. Included among these systems are prepaid group practices, like the Group Health Cooperative of Puget Sound and the Kaiser Permanente Medical Program, and prominent multi-specialty group practices, such as the Palo Alto Medical Clinic, the St. Louis Park Medical Center, and the Mayo Clinic.

Another way to reduce costs is to shorten the length of hospital stays for many conditions. For example, the standard length of stay for an uncomplicated myocardial infarction used to be three weeks. In the early 1970s randomized controlled trials, conducted at Massachusetts General Hospital, compared outcomes for patients hospitalized three weeks with those hospitalized for two weeks. No discernible differences were found.

A fifth way to cut costs is through simple cost-consciousness. Do not duplicate diagnostic workups. Use unit medical records, so that tests and histories are not repeated unnecessarily. Use outpatient surgical facilities. Of course, the key to all of these methods is the physician. While the gross incomes of physicians account for only about 18 percent of total health care spending, physicians' decisions control, or strongly influence, some 70 percent of total spending. Physicians order tests, recommend surgery, admit and discharge patients and the like. Thus, a sensible strategy to control health care costs is to enlist physicians as cost-effective managers of the health care system. It should be interesting and rewarding for physicians to develop organizations to reduce costs without cutting the quality of care. Some organized systems of care already manage to deliver good quality care at a considerably lower cost than average by using the cost-cutting techniques previously described. Hal Luft, of Stanford, reviewed the literature on health maintenance organizations (HMOs) and found that HMOs can take care of patients for ten to forty percent less cost per capita than the insured fee-for-service system. Studies of Medicare populations have yielded similar results.

One of the striking things about the health care sector is the variety of ways people have found to organize and to build in incentives for economy. Prepaid group practice is the largest single type of alternative delivery system, but it is definitely not the only model. In California and other states, individual practice associations preserve the solo, fee-for-service practice for those physicians and patients who prefer it, while at the same time, give physicians a vehicle to work together to cut costs. Although individual practice associations have not usually been as effective as prepaid group practices in controlling costs, they could become more effective if participating physicians were sufficiently committed to cost control to make substantial changes in their practice patterns.

Another alternative system is a primary care network similar to the ones developed by Safeco Insurance Company of Seattle, the Wisconsin's Physicians Service, and HMO of Pennsylvania. Under this model, the primary care physician does office-based primary care for a fixed monthly retainer fee per patient and controls and is at risk for the patient's specialty and hospital care. In effect the physician acts as the general manager of the patient's care. While this model needs further development, it appears to be a promising means for bringing incentives for economy to the individual physician, especially in rural and thinly populated areas.

Another model is the health alliance concept developed by Paul Ellwood. Under this model, a group of physicians, such as those at the Palo Alto Medical Clinic, work with a traditional insurer to offer a limited provider insurance plan whereby physician services are covered when obtained from or through a participating physician. Physicians work in whatever way they think is appropriate to hold down costs while providing good care.

The point is that there are a variety of models which allow for flexibility in adapting concepts to local conditions. One model will not meet the needs of every community in the United States.

If it is true that organized systems with built-in incentives for economy can deliver quality care at less cost, how can the number of these systems be increased? Government mandates are not the answer. Physicians and patients will not participate in an arrangement unless they perceive it to be compatible with their desire for good practice and quality care, i.e., it must be in both the physicians' and patients' best interest.

A means to achieve this goal is to create a framework in which those who would form and join economical systems of care can benefit from doing so through a system of fair economic competition among alternative health care financing and delivery organizations.

The principles of such a system are:

1.  Multiple choice. Once a year, or whatever period designated, each family is given a choice among competing health care financing and delivery plans operating in its community.

2.  Fixed dollar subsidies. Assistance given people from the government, from their employer, from Medicare or Medicaid, is in the form of a fixed dollar amount equal with respect to whichever plan is chosen. In this way, the family that chooses a more costly health care system pays more and, therefore, becomes cost conscious and motivated to seek out value for that extra payment.

3.  Rules of governance applied equally to all competitors. Rules are definitely needed to: (a) curb preferred risk selection, that is to make sure that the health plans prosper by providing better care at less cost and not by skillfully avoiding the enrollment and care of people who are really sick; (b) prevent people from manipulating and taking advantage of the system to avoid paying for health insurance until they get sick; (c) prevent the selling of deceptive or inadequate coverage; and (d) govern financial solvency.

4.  Physicians organized in competing economic units. Limited or preferred provider plans are needed whereby a beneficiary signs up with one plan and agrees to receive care from or through the physicians participating in that plan. Open or closed panels can be used.

If a system operating under these four principles existed, people would seek out the delivery model that offered them good value and, as a consequence, the health care delivery system would be transformed gradually and voluntarily into one offering choice and value to consumers. The winners of the competition would be those that did a good job for their patients both from a medical and economic point of view.

Unfortunately these principles, for the most part, are not applied today. For example, even in Santa Clara County, where alternative systems are established and known, in 1979, 73 percent of employers with under 500 employees and 36 percent of employers with more than 500 employees did not offer their employees a choice of health plans.

The tax consequences of fixed dollar contributions may be one reason the development of new models is slow. Currently, most employers pay 100 percent of the cost of an employee's health insurance coverage. If the employer pays for the insurance, it is paid for with pretax dollars and not included in the employee's taxable income. If the employer gave the employee the money to buy his own insurance, the employee would be buying insurance with net-after-tax dollars which would nearly double the cost. This has become more and more important as inflation has pushed everyone into higher tax brackets. Thus tax laws enacted in a different era with a different purpose have an enormous effect on health care financing.

Another hinderance is that the medical profession has enforced the idea of free choice of physician which means that insurance premiums are the same whether a person goes to the most expensive or the most economical physician. As a result there is little price competition among physicians. It is neccessary to reinterpret the principle of free choice of physician so that first, people have a free choice among alternative delivery systems. Then they can choose among the physicians participating in that system.

There are governmental proposals on the national level to direct public policy toward the creation of fair economic competition. In 1977, I proposed to the Carter administration a Consumer Choice Health Plan based on the Federal Employees Health Benefits Plan. The closest legislative approximation to that plan was the National Health Care Reform bill introduced in June 1980 by Representatives Richard Gephardt of Missouri and David Stockman of Michigan.

The same principles can be applied on an incremental basis to modify the present system of health care finance, which is based mainly on employment. For example, Senator David Durenberger's Health Incentives Reform bill requires certain employers to offer choices in plans, limits the exclusion of employer contributions from employee taxable income, and provides uniform minimum standards applicable to all of the tax favored health plans. A similar bill, the Health Cost Restraint Act, was introduced in 1979 by Representative Al Ullman, then Chairman of the House Ways and Means Committee. Representative Ullman's bill mandated a statewide demonstration of Project Health, a model in Multnomah County, Oregon for financing medical care for the poor through a system of competing private health care plans.

Another timely idea was recommended by the Health Policy Advisory Group to President-elect Reagan and is a phased Medicare reform plan modeled after the Federal Employees Health Benefits Plan. Medicare is based on the principles of cost reimbursement and fee-for-service, and therefore, systematically pays more for people who choose more costly systems and styles of care. The law, which is incredibly complex and has been revised over 2,600 times, is about 140 pages long; the regulations are more than 400 pages of

fine print; and the provider manual has some 700 pages. By com-
parison, the Federal Employees Health Benefits Plan law has eight
pages; the regulations are 16 pages; and the provider manual has
about 100 pages. The basis of the plan is that the federal government provides a formula of how much it will contribute. The
employee then picks a program from several choices. The market,
not complicated regulations, polices the system.

Using this system, the government could translate its present out-
lay per capita for Medicare into fixed dollar amounts, adjusted
yearly for inflation. Then the Health Care Financing Adminstration
could contract in each state with health insurers and health maintenance organizations to offer a comprehensive private sector
health care plan to Medicare beneficiaries. Every year enrollees
could designate the plan of their choice and the government would
contribute its fixed amount to the plan, with excess premium costs,
if any, paid for by the enrollee. This could be a very important
and valuable step forward, and would greatly simplify the administration and financing of health care under Medicare.

Focusing on the state level, a sensible strategy for Tennessee
would have two major components: the creation of the conditions
for fair market competition, and the creation of competitors. With
respect to creating conditions for a fair market, the idea is to
expand the number of people who have choices of health plans and
a fixed dollar contribution from either employers or the government. There are various ways to do this. In California, state
employees receive health benefits in a plan similar to the federal
employees plan. Discussion is now going on to extend this plan
to additional California public sector employees. Unfortunately,
local governments and unions are still more interested in using
health insurance plans for their own bargaining purposes than in
helping to create a competitive market beneficial to all.

Another approach is Oregon's Project Health which serves as a
broker to respond to the need for aggregate purchasing power. A
problem for small employers is to make their plans economical and
effective, and Project Health provides one means to accomplish
this.

A third approach is through private sector employers. This is the
approach used in Minneapolis/St. Paul and in Hawaii. In Hawaii,
virtually all of the employers now offer a choice between Hawaii
Medical Services Association and the Kaiser Permanente Medical Program. The result has been cost-effective care as evidenced by the
fact that hospital costs per capita in Hawaii are about two-thirds
of the national average, while the cost of living in general is
about 20 percent above the national average. Similarly, in northern California, a growing number of employers are following the
example of Hewlett Packard and Stanford University and adopting
the principle that their employees should have choices on an economically fair basis.

As to the problem of creating competitors, there is no simple or
single formula, but some ideas have been successfully tried elsewhere. One is to find or create a multi-specialty group that is

more economical and efficient than the average, and for that group to either create its own financing vehicle or to contract with an insurance company.  This was essentially the strategy of the Palo Alto Medical Clinic and of the St. Louis Park Medical Center.  Another approach is for employers to ask an insurer to create a limited provider plan with incentives for economy.  For example, in northern California, the telephone company played a key role in the creation of the United Medical Clinic's prepaid plan, the predecessor of the Take Care HMO.

A third approach is for a health center such as The University of Tennessee Center for the Health Sciences to sponsor a health care system, as have Harvard and Georgetown Universities.  However, the experiences of both would suggest that it is much tougher for universities to establish successful programs than might be anticipated.  Thus, if this approach is tried, it is important that persons with good business backgrounds participate in the development and operation of the system.

A final comment is that there are a vast number of proposals for health care cost control which I would call "tinkering," things like co-payments, people being paid for not going to the doctor, second opinions and fee schedules.  I do not see any evidence that these "tinkering" schemes can have a significant long-term, cost-reducing impact.  The real economy in health care will come through the growth of efficiently organized systems of care which are given a fair chance to compete.

Let me caution that competition is not a panacea.  It will not be easy or work quickly.  It is a slow-acting, long-term remedy which will take effort and commitment.  But experience shows that it can succeed and that is more than can be said for any other approach that is likely to be acceptable in the United States.

# RESPONSE
## Robert A. Derzon

In my copy of the book <u>Health Plan:  The Only Practical Solution to</u> <u>the Costs of Medical Care</u>, there is an author's inscription:

> "To Bob Derzon, the last of the great health regulators, with my esteem and affection."  Alain Enthoven

I intend to respond to Dr. Enthoven's thesis by pointing out some of its blessings, problems and impacts, and to amplify it by describing complementary strategies that must accompany any program to expand competition.  I also expect to perhaps puncture a few holes in his California warm air balloon by expanding the critical dialogue his challenging ideas present.

Lest there are any doubts about my reaction, I will give you my conclusions first and then attempt to explain them. Like Dr. Enthoven, I advocate competition, consumer choice, lower health care costs and private sector initiatives.  But there are severe obstacles--political, philosophical and technical--that have to be overcome to achieve these objectives.

Government experience has taught me an important lesson which is that the higher health care costs rise, the more dependent Americans become on public financing for the vulnerable, the poor, the aged and the sick.  Unfortunately, the higher the public bill, the greater the risk of cutbacks in service to those most in need, the greater the government inclination to regulate and the larger the leverage of public funds on the private delivery system.  The issues of affordability and cost are an absolutely critical baseline for both buyers and sellers of health care services.  Dr. Enthoven's diagnosis of the industry's cost inducing behavior is accurate but I remain less confident than he that the single strategy of competition is a sufficient remedy.

Some blessings of the Enthoven strategy are:

1.    The plan stresses incentives for good patient care while forcing providers and consumers to think through the extravagance, or at

21

least the price, of flat-of-the curve medicine, i.e., low marginal yield medicine. Today, there are very few market pressures to dampen the public's appetite for unlimited blank check health care services.

2.    The plan encourages the development of group practice and prepayment--two old ideas that when performed well can truly help patients, particularly the elderly who need convenience and comprehensive services, and the chronically ill who need medical continuity.

3.    The plan addresses a long overdue problem--runaway tax subsidies which tend to be a bigger benefit to higher paid employees than to lower paid workers. This regressive tax loophole either should be eliminated or capped because these expenditures are a hidden expense of government as foregone revenues. Tax subsidies currently for the young, the wealthy and the healthy equal over 50 percent of Medicare costs.

4.    The plan has awakened private industry and big labor to the costs and inequities of the fringe benefit for health insurance, and to the fact that industry can and should be a potent force for cost control and organization reform.

5.    The plan offers beneficial features such as a basic minimum benefit package, a cap on the tax subsidy, and gap filling requirements for private insurance including coverage for dependents and for employees between work periods.

6.    The plan, if applied to federal beneficiaries, could ease significantly the government's administrative burdens. As a result, the government's principal issues could become ones of protecting against anti-competitive behavior, assuring quality of health plans and setting reasonable capitation rates.

7.    The plan, over time, presents powerful incentives to use hospitals sparingly. That could be a plus or minus in the eyes of many in the health care field, but on balance, improved appropriate utilization of hospital services is a goal all should welcome.

8.    The plan to the extent that it strengthens the private sector, will have the positive effect of minimizing government responsibility and returning responsibility to the private sector where it belongs.

Notwithstanding these blessings, there are powerful transitional problems in any move to a competitive mode. It is unimaginable that over the next few years, even with legislative stimulation, the American health system can dramatically change deeply rooted values, cherished professional traditions, and long established relationships between physicians and patients. The Enthoven plan has risks and to a degree, unresolved problems. Many critics challenge its basic assumptions and question certain conclusions. I also have some concerns:

1.    The poor and aged sick will be left out because there is little

evidence that competing health organizations will go after the expensive and hard to take care of patients. There may be competition, but every indication is that very strong safeguards must be built in to protect access for those who are vulnerable and sick. A relatively small number of patients account for a very large percentage of costs in conventional health insurance and Medicare and Medicaid programs, and thus skew health costs. Keeping these patients out can be very advantageous to competing health plans. Without safeguards the Consumer Choice Plan could be relabeled the Provider Choice Plan with each plan making its own choices through skillful marketing or the strategic location of services and facilities.

2.    Competition is not easily developed, particularly in fields which tend to be natural monopolies. The Twin Cities, in presenting several alternate health delivery organizations, is still an exception and not the rule. Moreover, even where prepaid practice is highly developed, such as in the San Francisco Bay area, competition is not assured. Physicians are the key to building alternative health systems. They must be willing to take financial risks with their daily medical practices. However, as long as generous fee-for-service arrangements exist, many physicians will refuse to gamble on capitation. Moreover, even where there is a willingness to change, management expertise and to some extent capital formation to operate new modes of care are still in short supply.

3.    Competition among health plans may not bring down prices, at least not rapidly. Some critics believe that although hospital days per 1000 subscribers in health plans are lower than for equivalent persons in the fee-for-service market, the savings may be simply pocketed by the plan through physician bonuses, new building funds or rainy day funds. These same critics argue that premiums of some health plans are priced up to the bottom of the fee-for-service market because most members select their plan based on convenience of the physician's office and not on the cost of the plan. Research shows that although health maintenance organization (HMO) costs are ten to forty percent less than traditional medical care costs for the same services on age adjusted populations, HMO costs in many locations appear to be rising at about the same rate as the non-HMO sector. This is not an argument against competition and choice, but rather an argument that costs may not be substantially less, at least not in the early years.

4.    Business and labor may not be willing to change their collective bargaining agreements. Equal employer payment for each worker's health benefit is such an obvious and equitable solution that it is difficult to imagine workers demanding less. Yet at Chrysler, where the last contract negotiated $1.17 an hour for health benefits, the contract promised service benefits to workers and their families. Management pays the full cost which is about $140.00 a month to Kaiser or $202.00 a month to Blue Cross. Management would probably argue to average the existing cost, perhaps at $165.00 a month. This means that suddenly the autoworker on Blue Cross must pay $37.00 a month out-of-pocket to

preserve his same level of benefits. In turn, the autoworker in Kaiser believes management owes him $25.00 a month, the difference between the average employer contribution of $165.00 and the Kaiser cost.   It is arguments on these issues that stifle legislative initiatives as even a worthy Enthoven idea could mean the loss of hard won benefits to individual workers.

In addition to the above problems, several key questions need to be addressed. What does an employer do when he cannot find alternative health plans to offer his employees? What do multi-plant employers do about health care cost differences among the several regions in which they manufacture goods or distribute services? How are health plans made to include genuine open enrollment, while not discriminated against because of "community" rating of premiums? How can competing plans be made to offer a decent range of basic health benefits so that prices can be compared for the same product?

Most of these issues can be answered by law and regulation so that in a sense we are not discussing "competition versus regulation." Many of these tough questions have been answered by Dr. Enthoven but not to the satisfaction of those large constituency groups-- politicians, big business, labor unions, insurance industry and organized medicine--needed to have a successful legislative course. These large public constituencies must be developed for a legislative thrust toward competition to be successful.

The impact of competition on hospitals, physicians and medical schools must also be considered, and with a brief preliminary cautionary comment, I will indulge in the liberty of forecasting the possible consequences for these groups.

The caution is that initially impact will largely be a function of the following equation:

> The market share of the population which enrolls in com-
> peting plans plus the willingness of government at both
> the state and federal level to provide more attractive
> financing for public beneficiaries who could be enrolled
> plus the number and size of competing plans in a region.

Assuming these factors are significant, I will speculate that hospitals will be faced with the following:

- Direct and tougher negotiations with private health plans than with current purchasers.

- Government demands for the same discounts private insurers obtain.

- Fewer days of hospital care per 1000.

- High cost hospitals in a non-preferred position, although there will always be a nucleus of the population who will not be price sensitive.

- Some hospitals and their medical staffs becoming a health plan and marketing a full range of services.

- Costly technology more easily regionalized.

- More hospital mergers and consolidations occurring to gain seller negotiating power, reduce duplicate health services and more easily close beds.

- Grave trouble for teaching and community hospitals providing unreimbursed services to the poor.

The impact of a genuinely competitive market on physicians suggests that:

- New physicians will seek out the safety and convenience of an already assembled medical practice.

- Primary care physicians will be strategically advantaged in the gatekeeper role.

- Large proportions of physicians will be salaried with incentives in multi-disciplinary group practices.

- Rates of surgical intervention will be reduced.

- Some medical technologies will lose their glamour.

- Surgeons' incomes will more closely approximate internists' incomes.

- Physicians will retain a larger share of the health dollar, a dollar which may expand somewhat more slowly in the future.

The prospects for medical schools and medical centers do not seem particularly heartening in this brave new world of competition.  I suggest these possibilities:

- A loss of certain insurable patients who will seek routine bread and butter care elsewhere.

- The chance that medical centers will shirttail alternative delivery systems for their tertiary care.

- A drive to identify medical education costs and discontinue their financing through sick funds.

- An even more emphatic demand for primary care physician training in lieu of specialty and sub-specialty preparation.

- Depending upon the development of vouchers for the poor and near poor, the possible loss of the traditional market of indigent patients.

- Some very genuine pressures to increase educational and clinical efficiencies in the university hospital setting.

- A re-examination, and in fact retreat, by some community hospital affiliates of their health profession education and training programs.

Since I do not believe that competition is going to occur overnight, even in a totally hospitable environment, concurrent strategies must be found to complement those of consumer choice. I believe that industry and individuals can contribute to constrain health care costs. Furthermore, government has an extra obligation to redirect public policy so that health expenditures do not outdistance its tax revenues and trust fund income over the next few years.

Like it or not, government is now purchasing close to 55 percent of nursing home and hospital services, and 18 percent of physician services. Government can and must become a more effective purchaser of health services. This will not be easy because of the classical values on which principles of government rest. These values of social insurance protection and security, the promised entitlement of health services rather than of indemnity dollars, and free choice of providers are among the very root causes of the surge in health care costs.

Government cannot sit still, nor should it, with respect to public policy initiatives. The new administration, while contemplating competition, should move foward to allow:

1.    Prospective hospital payment with efficiency incentives that are firm and predictable.

2.    Easing of payment restrictions for public beneficiary programs that pertain to capitation so that public beneficiaries can choose among a greater range of health providers including willing HMOs.

3.    The replacement of UCR, an inflationary and inequitable physician payment program, with more rigorous assignment terms and a decent fee schedule.

4.    Modification of free choice of provider perhaps through beneficiary incentives.

5.    Joining of governments with private buyers to negotiate terms with sellers of health services.

6.    A temporary constraint on capital flow into the health market until marketplace competition takes hold.

Without complementary strategies for government purchases, plans for a more competitive health system seem even more remote. Therefore, I do applaud Alain Enthoven's bold approaches, while raising several of the major obstacles to implementation, speculating on some impacts which may be generalized, and suggesting that government move in tandem.

The Enthoven concepts are perhaps the most provocative and indeed among the most imaginative ideas to surface in U.S. health policy in the last decade. They have the attraction and the special quality of allowing for a heavy dose of private sector initiative and response in an era in which disillusionment and frustration with government policy in health care and health care financing is running rampant. They deserve thoughtful discussion and debate.

# III
# THE CALIFORNIA EXPERIENCE
# Robert D. Burnett

For the employed individual in California, marketplace solicitation of his enrollment in various health care delivery systems is nearly an accomplished fact. The competition, for a variety of reasons, has not yet become involved with the Medicare or Medicaid systems, but as competition expands and its physician members continue to expand, it is inevitable that competition will involve the governmentally funded sector. Presently in California, approximately 20 percent of the population (about four million people) are enrolled in a prepaid plan of a health maintenance organization (HMO) or alternative delivery system (ADS) type. When one considers the number of people in the state on Medicare (15 percent) and Medicaid (14 percent) coupled with the HMO and ADS enrollment, only 50 percent of Californians are not enrolled in one of these programs. This 50 percent is being vigorously solicited to join various plans in many areas of the state.

The earliest significant ADS plan was the Ross-Loos Clinic in Los Angeles, founded about 50 years ago. It was followed by the famous Kaiser Permanente Plan which had its earliest origins in the state of Washington in 1933 and was first offered in California in 1942. Particularly in their early years, Kaiser and Ross-Loos relied heavily on organized labor for their growth. The growth of Kaiser has been particularly remarkable, as currently there are about 3.2 million people enrolled in Kaiser, equally split between the plans in northern and southern California. Kaiser's annual dollar volume of business is around $1.5 billion. Perhaps, even more significant is the fact that in northern California about one out of every two employees offered the option of joining the Kaiser plan does so.

About 20 years ago, partially to meet the competitive threat and partially out of a feeling of social responsibility, about half of the non-rural county medical associations in California developed foundations for medical care. These foundations

27

offered the indemnity insurance companies a mechanism which would conduct peer review, process both inpatient and out-patient claims, and guarantee that participating physicians would not charge over the maximum fee schedule or balance bill the patient. In return, the medical foundations required the insurance companies to meet certain specifications of coverage (viz., not excluding newborn coverage from the time of birth) and thus avoided the typically evolving Swiss cheese health insurance package of a decade ago. In these foundations, physicians were not at risk. Although the foundations attracted significant portions of the market, between ten and twenty percent of the total population in the Sacramento, San Jose and San Diego areas, and created a climate of restraint on length of stay and physician over-utilization, they did not and still do not have comprehensive benefits, provider incentives or the integrated system approach necessary for effective marketplace competition to the continued expansion of the Kaiser closed panel system.

From the foundations, there has recently evolved a series of broad-based independent practice associations (IPA) which uti-lize the foundation expertise in peer review and claims processing. The IPAs are open to most of the members of the medical society who wish to participate and enter into direct market competition with the Kaiser system and the various other closed panel systems functioning in California. Presently, six of these organizations are federally qualified HMOs, and two more broad-based IPAs are in the process of qualifying.

The basic method for funding an IPA varies considerably. The oldest of these in Sacramento relied on government grants. Lifeguard in Santa Clara County, in an effort to promote cost containment and cost awareness in the hospital sector, required a $100,000 contribution from each hospital to participate. This was an effort to provide an incentive to the hospitals to make the plan a marketplace success which success partially depends on cost constraint and efficiency of the hospital delivery system. Funds raised from participating physicians were also a source of capital for the Lifeguard IPA. In San Diego County, the principal funding came from the physicians involved with initial fees of $500 required for participation; the fee is now over $1000. These broad-based IPAs cover all the metropolitan marketplace areas of California except for Los Angeles and Orange Counties.

It is interesting to note that the employer climate in California is such that most of the major employers are requiring federal certification before an HMO plan is offered to their employees. Thus, all of the plans that are expanding to any degree are federally qualified.

In contrast to the rest of California, Los Angeles, the most populous area of the state, never had a medical care foundation. This perhaps accounts for the lack of development of a broad-based IPA. In 1972, the Reagan administration stim-ulated the development of primary health care plans (PHP) for

Medicaid recipients. Unfortunately, many of the plans qualified under the state statutes were poorly organized, had poor managers, and at times engaged in a skimming process to enroll only healthy people. In addition, many had barriers to care for the MediCal population they enrolled. The deficiencies in these plans stimulated the growth of extremely restrictive state regulations for prepaid plans, regulations far stricter and difficult to qualify under than the federal HMO laws. Nevertheless, a certain number of these PHPs function well and have expanded and become federally qualified. Several of the PHPs that are not federally qualified still deal only with Medicaid recipients and are fairly stagnant in their growth pattern. These plans are mainly group or staff model plans.

Currently, there are 32 HMOs functioning in California, of which 21 are federally qualified. Of these, as far as can be determined, six have their origins from foundations of medical care; two are network plans; one is Blue Cross of Northern California; one is Blue Cross of Southern California; two are the Kaiser plans of northern and southern California; four were originally hospital inspired or hospital based; one was developed by a county government; one was developed by the Safeco Insurance Company; and 12 survived from the PHP concept.

A major competitive mechanism in California in the HMO field is Blue Cross. In northern California, Blue Cross initially developed a pilot project in conjunction with the foundation in Santa Clara County. This pilot project was eminently successful and was the forerunner of the present broad-based Lifeguard IPA. The program was marketed to 3000 people. In the initial step, Blue Cross assumed the risk for the costs of hospitalization, and the physicians assumed the risk for the medical costs or non-hospital costs of the plan. A risk withhold of 15 percent was withheld from physician's fees as an incentive to deter over-utilization. A maximum fee schedule was allowed. The plan operated experimentally for two years, during which time it was able to pay back the risk factor to the physicians, as well as allow Blue Cross to break even.

As mentioned previously, the employers in Santa Clara County insisted that any plan be federally qualified before they offered it to their employees. With that in mind, the physicians in the Foundation sat down at the negotiating table with Blue Cross and attempted to work out the organizational structure for an HMO. It soon became clear to the physicians that the power and control of the organization would be at Blue Cross headquarters in Oakland, California. This was unacceptable to the physicians, just as physician control was unacceptable to Blue Cross. Consequently, negotiations broke off. At that juncture, Blue Cross began to form its own closed panel network to compete in the HMO market in northern California. They had pilot projects with four large excellent multi-specialty clinics, three in Santa Clara County and one in the contiguous county of San Mateo. This HMO was qualified as an IPA although physicians looked at it as a group plan because membership was open only to physicians participating full time in one of the four multi-specialty clinics. The reason for the entrance of Blue Cross in the marketplace as an IPA is quite obvious. The dual choice section of the HMO law allowed Blue Cross to offer the plan to employers as an IPA in a dual choice option with Kaiser, and thus not be in the position where the employer could choose Kaiser over the Blue Cross IPA model, as might occur if Blue Cross offered a group model that would allow each employee the choice between Kaiser and Blue Cross.

At about the same time that Blue Cross was organizing its closed panel IPA, which had expanded to involve several other multi-specialty clinics in northern California, the physicians were reorganizing and trying to raise funds to develop an IPA in Santa Clara County. Concomitantly, in southern California, Blue Cross was developing a Health Network which did not necessarily rely on multi-specialty groups but did rely upon groups of physicians to be its members. The Network has grown very fast and is approaching 100,000 members.

Another important development in the HMO field in California is the purchase of established HMOs by large corporations. Insurance Company of North America purchased Ross-Loos which is now functioning as an IPA. In addition, INA has another HMO in southern California and is making overtures to buy one of the certified HMOs in northern California which had evolved from a prepaid Medicaid-type plan. There is other evidence in California of large corporate interest in buying HMO plans in order to use their license to expand into the competitive marketplace force. Whether the entrance of the corporate insurance conglomerates into the HMO field will lead to a situation in which they market their plans as a loss leader, utilize reserves to capture the marketplace, force out competition and, thus, have a better chance later to increase their premium rates, remains to be seen. But this is a distinct possibility.

The Safeco plan, a non-federally qualified plan originated by Safeco Insurance Company of Seattle, is another classic model. It functions in Woodland, California and has about 14,000 enrollees. Safeco uses a primary care model with two risk pools, one for the primary physician and one for all the medical and hospital expenses that the patient engenders outside of the primary care physician. The patient must go to the primary physician first or be authorized by him to see another doctor. The funds for the non-primary physician come out of the second risk pool. If money is left over in this pool, the insurance plan splits it with the primary care physician. If the pool is used up, some of the primary physician's capitation money is refunded to the plan. Under this model, the entire control of medical care delivery rests in the hands of the primary physician who also is responsible for coordinating the expenditure of medical funds. Many believe that although putting the management of the patient under the proper type of physician is a move in the right direction, it is an over-correction of a problem in the indemnity model where patients go from specialist to specialist.

All the IPA-HMOs of a broad-based nature or to some extent the foundation-type plans use the primary physician model. In the Santa Clara plan, each member is required to designate a primary physician and the ability to see one of the participating specialists in the plan depends upon authorization from the primary physician. The degree to which this rule is enforced varies greatly from one plan to another. The Santa Clara plan is less stringent than many other plans because it realizes it is often more efficacious for a person with a visual problem to go directly to the ophthalmologist. In the Blue Cross Take Care plan, capitation is firmer. The multi-specialty clinic which is capitated assumes the medical risk and Blue Cross assumes the hospital risk. The clinic, in turn, often capitates their primary physicians by giving them so much per month and also provides a secondary pool, much as in the Safeco plan, for the specialist physicians within the clinic. This type of arrangement is followed by the large, rather well known Palo Alto Medical Clinic.

There are other models that have been developed in California. There is the hospital-based HMO in which one hospital with a group of physicians develops an HMO. There is a plan in which a public group usually in conjunction with a portion of the medical society develops a plan. Finally, there is one plan which was developed under the auspices of the county government as a PHP plan. This plan is now trying to expand into the private market, but is still controlled by the county government.

Obviously, in California, the structure for competition has evolved and is in place, and the number of people enrolled in these plans is increasing rapidly. Although Kaiser is by far the dominant factor, the growth rate of many of the newer plans is phenomenal. Within its first six months, the plan in San Diego County was able to enroll 20,000 people. So it is very likely that in many areas of California significant competition will continue between various health care delivery systems.

To be more specific about the nuts and bolts of competition, honed down to a local area, the development of the plan in Santa Clara County will be described. Santa Clara County, a prosperous county of 1.2 million people, is endowed with over 1600 practicing physicians, not including the physicians at Stanford Medical Center or at a large Veterans Hospital facility. As previously noted, when the negotiations for forming an HMO broke off between Blue Cross and the Foundation it behooved the physicians to raise the funds to establish their own IPA. It was ascertained that to be reasonably operable it would take about a half million dollars. As those involved in this field know, to be federally qualified a plan must have a functioning and in place marketing staff, financial staff and executive directorship. This requires money and time. The physicians did not conduct a feasibility study or apply for federal grants, but did collect $100,000 from each participating hospital plus membership fees from physicians.

It was not terribly difficult to convince the physicians in the county to participate in the plan. At the time of the plan's development, there was a closed panel, federally qualified plan in the county, propped up by federal grant money, which grew from 3000 to 30,000 people in one year. The plan was really run by people with no experience in the medical care field and was offered to subscribers at a cost considerably less than the Kaiser Permanente plan, although the benefit package had to be the same. Needless to say, the plan had rapid growth and was soon in the red. This occurred shortly after the physicians plan became federally qualified. Nonetheless, in the development stage of raising the money, the physicians in the county were faced with the fact that closed panel medicine was growing at a rate of 25 percent per year. If extrapolated out, that meant that no patients would be left in the private sector in six and one-half years. Of course it is unlikely that any one system would dominate the marketplace to the exclusion of all the others, but this certainly pointed out the need for physicians to become involved in a competing HMO.

Once the money was raised the problem was to become federally qualified. Approval was delayed while the federal government tried to rescue the ailing plan described above. This set back the physicians plan in the marketplace to the extent that Blue Cross was able to become qualified closely after it. Thus the physicians plan had no real jump in the marketplace over its competition. The physicians plan competes with Kaiser, a closed panel, efficient, well-funded, well-established plan with a good reputation. It also competes with a closed panel series of clinics which essentially deliver care at three major places in the county and have a great deal of peer pressure to control utilization. These clinics are capitated in much the same way as the Kaiser Permanente Medical plans are capitated. The physicians plan does not control the appointment book in the manner that Kaiser does. That is, if someone calls up the Kaiser plan and states he has a sore throat, the nurse may well say that most sore throats are viral and will be gone in a few days, so it probably is not necessary to come in, but if you stay sick, then come in. Whereas, under the physicians plan, if a patient calls and wants to see the doctor, 99 percent of the time the request is granted. Therefore, access to care is not limited in the same fashion, and premiums, of necessity, must be somewhat higher. To balance higher premiums, there is a wider choice of physicians. Two of the three multi-specialty clinics involved in the Take Care plan also participate in the physicians plan with the result that it has an even wider choice of medical care systems.

Having the highest premium leads to a certain degree of adverse selection which depends on the out-of-pocket contribution by the employee. Aware of this, the plan avoids like the plague employers who make small contributions to their employees health benefits package because if contributions are small, the difference of maybe $15 per month between the plan and Kaiser's plan, all but sick people are precluded from participating. Many of the employers in the county, however, do offer rather generous health benefit plans and the differentials are not too great. However, the amount of the out-of-pocket cost that the employee must contribute to the plan he joins can be significant. An interesting comparison of plans in the county is that the Palo Alto Medical Clinic's portion of the Take Care plan is about 227 days per 1000 whereas the physicians plan has approximately 377 days and Kaiser about 390 per 1000. Thus, hospitalization is pared down to the bare bones level with most of the funds of the enrollees going for outpatient medical and laboratory care.

There are many other things that occur in a competitive situation such as the one in California. In the closed panel plan, particularly in the closed panel Kaiser plan, people in primary practice see on the average of about one Kaiser patient per day. With about 500 non-Kaiser physicians in the county seeing one Kaiser patient per day, Kaiser would be allowed to reduce its premium $10 million per year in the county. That is the same as a subsidization of $3 million a year in the county for their plan. This subsidization is in no way reciprocated in the physicians plan since no one enrolled in the plan is allowed to go outside of it and still receive benefits. Of course, since every type of service is available in the plan, there really is no reason to go outside.

As to physician involvement in the plan, physicians certainly demonstrated considerable concern for the plan's success. However, it is difficult for a physician to alter his style of practice for the two or three percent of the people that are in the plan and for which he is at a financial risk. Practice patterns change slowly. This does, however, have a ripple effect on other indemnity plans for it promotes cost awareness within the county.

Anticipatory peer review guidelines for various specialties are developed by the specialist members of the plan. For example, in pediatrics there is an outline of the permissible number of well-child visits and the type of care that should be rendered at each. In addition, the maximum amount of laboratory and other ancillary tests allowed for various age groups are listed. There is a pre-admission hospital certification which in some specialties is quite strict. For instance, obstetrician-gynecologists in the county decided that the indication for hysterectomy under the plan, other than exsanguination, was pre-admission certification by an obstetric-gynecologic representative.

The plan has done well in market penetration, in spite of the competition. But, there is no way to really compare patient encounters per plan members with other plans. Certainly, this is probably one of the most basic measures of such prepaid plans. Those that limit access to care too much may have a hospital utilization figure that is about the same as those who do not limit access to care, perhaps because some of their people get sicker. But limiting access certainly will show up in the number of patient encounters per physician per year.

Initial penetration of employees of a given organization varies primarily with:  (1) their past experience with a previously failed HMO; (2) the amount of time allowed by the employer, if any, for presentation to employees; (3) the differential between the plans offered and the indemnity plan of the employer; and (4) the general attitude of the employer toward this movement.  In spite of what appears in the newspapers or some of the trade magazines, many national employers, who give lip service to the HMO movement, are very restrictive in their acceptance of it within their own plants.  In Santa Clara County, this problem may be due to local resistance and the fact that to some extent the workload of the benefits manager is increased if more than one plan is available to employees.

The physicians plan has been operational for over a year and has a growth rate that is slow but steady.  The plan is very selective in its offerings in order to accumulate adequate data on utilization and avoid marked adverse risk selection.  There has been excellent growth of new people coming to work for employers to whom the plan is already available, and in the few plants that have come around to offering the plan a second time the penetration rates have greatly increased.  It is not uncommon to have an initial penetration rate of only two to four percent.  In essence, the plan seems to be marketed very well by word of mouth of the employees within a given organization.  There have been very few defections from the plan.  Of the nearly 900 physicians who joined the plan, only two have resigned.  Although the plan has a federal loan to use to supplement its private initial capital sources, it has drawn on the loan fund considerably less than projected and within a year repayment will begin.

Success has been achieved in spite of vigorous competition and I think it is dependent upon the plan's excellent management, the perceptiveness of its actuarial firm, and the commitment of the physicians involved.  The plan is making adequate strides to develop an alternative system that does not drastically limit access to care or decrease the quality of care available. Even though large fiscal reserves are allied against the plan it is growing well, doing better financially than anticipated, and securing a greater commitment from the physicians in the county than initially expected.  The plan fully intends to be the dominant health care delivery organization in Santa Clara County.

# RESPONSE
# Thomas E. Nesbitt

The California experience, described by Dr. Burnett, indicates a number of diverse issues worthy of consideration. The issue of competition itself must be thoroughly analyzed as it implies a realignment of incentives in health care. The manner in which this realignment will affect the behavior patterns of consumers, physicians and hospital personnel is not very well understood, although it has been and continues to be the object of considerable study and conjecture.

Competitive activity is one method for allocating scarce resources, as contrasted to voluntary mechanisms and government regulation. The precise distribution of resources will, however, be influenced by a balance of all three of these mechanisms; that is voluntary, regulatory and competitive forces. Looking at some of the elements of competition, one can conclude that competition occurs at many levels within the health care system. At the first level, it appears as insurance companies compete with one another and with alternative delivery systems for enrollees. At the second level, it occurs as physicians compete for patients with other physicians and with alternative delivery systems. Given the coming physician surplus, this element will become increasingly acute. At the third level, hospitals compete with one another for patients.

At each of these levels, many factors influence the nature of the competition. For example, consumer choices are influenced by the fees charged by individual physicians, the convenience of receiving care from a specific physician or hospital, their perception of the quality of care to be rendered, and their perception of their own health status. Consumer choices of an insurance plan will similarly be influenced by its effects as it relates to these factors.

Physician utilization of hospital services in treating a patient is influenced principally by two sets of factors. First, the decision to admit is influenced by the patient's condition and clarity of symptoms, and the physician's own training experience and attitude towards other forms of treatment. Second, the decision

35

is influenced by the availability of hospital beds and resources as determined by the hospital's perception of its role and the hospital's recognition of community needs and physician and consumer demands. All of these elements are a part of the competitive picture and must be integrated and analyzed.

An analysis of these elements must include a study of the way they relate to the role of insurance. In addition, it is necessary to investigate the effect of competitive mechanisms created by employer activities and by government activities through regulatory and tax policies.

The consumer choice approach discussed by Dr. Enthoven rests on several critical assumptions: (1) consumers will respond to differences in price, selecting lower cost forms of insurance over more expensive forms; (2) other insurers will attempt to cut hospital utilization and costs in an effort to meet the premiums of health maintenance organizations; (3) lower hospital utilization rates observed in alternative delivery systems are a result of greater cost consciousness on the part of the system's management and providers; (4) hospitals will respond to pressures from insurers and alternative delivery systems to reduce their costs in order to obtain contracts for the delivery of care to program enrollees; and (5) physicians will respond to the need to keep premiums low by ordering less expensive forms of medical care for their patients.

As indicated by Dr. Burnett, the final answer as to the validity of these assumptions has not been reached. Therefore, it becomes critical that these assumptions be tested to determine the potential impact of a consumer choice plan or any other "pro-competition" realignment of incentives. Such a test should involve the observation and documentation of consumer, hospital and physician responses to incentives that approximate a competitive environment.

A second issue relating to behavior patterns of physicians which merits attention and further discussion concerns reimbursement arrangements, educational programs and designation of participating physicians. There are frequent references to the economic incentives under fee-for-service reimbursement and to an assumption that this automatically leads physicians to maximize the amount of care delivered.

Medical economists view the fee-for-service system as creating incentives for excessive utilization--excessive medical care. The trade-off, however, is substitution with a system that creates potential disincentives for adequate medical care services. There will always be abuse in any system, by some. But the question of a public policy giving preference to this trade-off model should be carefully examined. This becomes even more critical when viewed as a cost measure. Total physician reimbursement today constitutes some 13 to 15 percent of the total health care dollar. Significant further reductions can scarcely be expected by the substitution of any other kind of physician reimbursement mechanism. A far better approach may be to focus on that 70 percent of the health care dollar that is spent under the direction of the physi-

cian, as such an approach would seem to offer a far greater potential for cost-effectiveness.

A third issue for consideration relates to financing structure.
Many view health maintenance organizations(HMO), independent practice associations and other alternative delivery systems as basically modifications of prepaid medical care financing schemes.

As a search is conducted for a better methodology, it would seem
prudent to give high priority to one element of the financing structure that has never been adequately addressed--initial physician
involvement.   Currently, contractual arrangements exist between
consumers who purchase a health care insurance plan from an insurance company or alternative delivery system, such as an HMO with
contractual arrangements with hospitals.  But, until very recently
a satisfactory arrangement has never been developed wherein the physician initially assumes significant financial responsibility in
the planning, organization and administration of an alternative
delivery system.   This may very well be the missing link in the
circle, and a highly significant one that has long been ignored.
If properly developed, constructed and administered, it would
seem most likely to provide that mechanism for the development of
accountability of behavior patterns that is so necessary if there
is to be an impact on that 70 percent of health care expenditures
controlled by physicians in their decision-making capacity.  Such
incentives accomplished through voluntary participation and peer
review would seem to offer another mechanism for the creation of
a successful alternative delivery system.

A final issue prompted by Dr. Burnett's presentation is that these
creative, competitive strategies might conceivably, and rather easily, result in a stifling of innovation and technology purely on
the basis of cost saving.  Should the progressive dynamics of the
health care system as it is known today be arrested and a freezing
of the system occur, the United States might find itself in the im-
age of Great Britain and Canada where progress has virtually ceased.
Certainly those who fail to study history are doomed to repeat it,
and here the historical perspectives deserve very careful scrunity.
Americans do not want the product delivered 25 years from now in
the medical marketplace to be the same as it is today, anymore than
they want to revert to the product of 25 years ago.

# IV
# THE OREGON EXPERIENCE
## W.T. Johnston

My personal biases favor the private mainstream of medical care for everyone, including the low income person, the elderly, and those categories of people that our government seems to classify in peculiar ways, as if they are not quite real persons. Also, I believe that everyone deserves to be paid a reasonable fee, or a reasonable stipend, for their services; and therefore the use of the discounted fee-for-service system to serve the poor is really not to be tolerated if mainstream quality and access are to be preserved.

The basic tenets of the Project Health concept are consistent with these beliefs and developed as a result of a belief that the system of separate care should be reversed. Two important people involved in creating this system, who gave it the necessary political and system power bases, were Commissioner Donald E. Clark, now the Executive Officer of the County; and Dr. Hugh H. Tilson, who came to Multnomah County as the Assistant Health Officer in 1971 and later took over as Health Officer and Director of the Multnomah County Department of Human Services. I was employed by these men in September of 1972 to begin planning for Project Health. A chronology of the program and project events that resulted can be presented as follows.

Project Health Chronology

Until 1973, the county operated a County Hospital located on the campus of the University of Oregon Health Sciences Center just south of downtown Portland. The Center's teaching staff and students provided excellent physician service, but the Center's location was very inconvenient to many potential users. In addition, the care represented a separate system for the county's low income residents.

In 1973, the Oregon Legislature authorized a State takeover of the facility, freeing up $4.2 million in county funds for Project

39

Health.  With the conceptual idea of a "broker" organization which would "pool" and administer funds from several sources, Donald Clark set out to utilize the $4.2 million as seed money to purchase mainstream medical care for the working poor and to attract federal and state funds to meet the needs of the then estimated 41,000 county residents who were medically indigent; that is, those with earnings above the welfare level, but unable to purchase adequate health care.

In the spring of 1973, Project Health began contracting with private community hospitals and physicians on the basis of negotiated prospective per diem rates.

In August of 1974, Project Health began subsidizing the cost of in-hospital care for low income clients enrolling in Cascade Health Care, Inc., a health maintenance organization (HMO) funded by the Public Health Service's Family Health Center (FHC) program.

In the Fall of 1974, the Health Administrator of Health and Human Services (HHS) Region X designated Project Health as a National Health Insurance Model and awarded $100,000 to the county for development of a Medical Management Information System.

A step toward actualization of the "pooling" concept was made in August of 1975, when Multnomah County was awarded $387,000 to administer medical services for 5,600 low-income people enrolled in the Kaiser Foundation Health Plan through Section 330 of the Public Health Service Act.

Also in 1975, the county's Health Department decategorized its traditional public health clinics to create eight decentralized access centers which function to provide a front door to the health care delivery system, as well as care of last resort, facilitating access to care in the mainstream for the medically needy.

In January of 1976, Project Health implemented enrollment of the medically indigent into prepaid care with Kaiser Foundation Health Plan, Oregon Physicians' Service (Blue Shield), Cascade Health Care and the University of Oregon Health Sciences Center Family Practice Clinic.

In February 1976, Project Health implemented the Medicaid Demonstration Project which combined federal, state and local funds to cover up to 3,400 people by June of 1979.  This was another milestone in the "pooling of funds" concept development.

During July 1977, two additional prepaid health care plans were added:  Portland Metro Health, a federally qualified health maintenance organization, and OPS/Providence Hospital and Medical Center Health Plan, a combination designed to serve Project Health as well as the teaching programs at two local hospitals.

In August 1977, Project Health became the grantee for Project Dental Health, which is funded through a Public Health Service Section 330 grant and is operated by contract with the University of Oregon School of Dentistry.

As of July 1978, new contracts eliminated the waiting period for prepaid plan enrollment; that is, clients began receiving first day coverage.

As June 30, 1979, the end of the grant award period for the Medicaid Demonstration Project approached, an interim evaluation of the project indicated that while several key questions had been answered during the grant period, some substantive issues were only beginning to become visible.  Because the program had enrolled 2,400 people, and their continued medical benefits had to be considered, state and county officials applied for, and subsequently received from the Health Care Financing Administration, a continuation of the program to June 30, 1980.  This extension permitted the county and state to develop a revised demonstration proposal aimed at addressing the substantive issues raised in the interim evaluation.

On May 16, 1980, a Notice of Grant Award was signed by the Health Care Financing Administration approving the "Multnomah County Medically Needy Demonstration Project" for the period July 1, 1980 through June 30, 1981.  The award approved a budget of $3,134,670 and granted 14 waivers to federal regulations.

Demographics

The following tables present (1) a population profile of Multnomah County and (2) figures indicating health insurance and HMO enrollment in the Portland Metropolitan area.

Table 1:  POPULATION PROFILE OF MULTNOMAH COUNTY (1976 estimate)

|  | POPULATION | PERCENT |
|---|---|---|
| NON-POOR | 400,000 | 71.9% |
| MEDICARE | 75,000 | 13.5% |
| WELFARE (Categorically Needy) | 40,000* | 7.2% |
| NON-WELFARE BUT POOR: Medically Needy and Non-Categorical Indigent | 41,000 | 7.4% |
| TOTAL POPULATION | 556,000 | 100.0% |

*Includes about 4,000 Medicare Aged and Disabled.*

COMPETITION IN THE MARKETPLACE

Table 2:   HEALTH INSURANCE AND HMO ENROLLMENT IN THE PORTLAND
                   METROPOLITAN AREA (1976-1977)[1]

|  | ENROLLMENT | PERCENT |
|---|---|---|
| **INSURANCE:** | | |
| BLUE CROSS | 270,000 | 22.5% |
| BLUE SHIELD (OPS) | 160,000 | 13.3% |
| AETNA | 50,000 | 4.2% |
| OTHERS | 216,000 | 18.0% |
| TOTAL INSURANCE | 696,000 | 58.0% |
| | | |
| **HMOS:** | | |
| KAISER | 200,000 | 16.7% |
| PORTLAND METRO HEALTH | 10,000 | 0.8% |
| CASCADE | 10,000 | 0.8% |
| PHYSICIANS ASSOCIATION | | |
| OF CLACKAMAS COUNTY | 8,000 | 0.7% |
| TOTAL HMOS | 228,000 | 19.0% |
| | | |
| **OTHER:** | | |
| WELFARE (NON-KAISER) | 45,000 | 3.8% |
| MEDICARE | 75,000 | 6.2% |
| UNINSURED [2] | 156,000 | 13.0% |
| TOTAL OTHER | 276,000 | 23.0% |
| | | |
| **METROPOLITAN AREA TOTAL** | 1,200,000 | 100.0% |

[1]Federal Trade Commission, "The Health Maintenance Organization
and Its Effect on Competition," July 1977.

[2]Oregon Research Institute, Oregon Opinion Index, December 1975.

## Description of the Project in Terms of Its Principles

The ten basic principles around which Project Health was developed and is currently operating are:

1. **Mainstream medicine** for the Project's clients.

   The number one objective and principle of the Project Health concept is that each Project Health client should be given equal treatment for better or for worse.  He should be en- rolled in the same community health plans that are used by other individuals in the community.  In order to avoid the stigma of being poor and indigent, Project Health's clients are very difficult to identify, as once enrolled in a health plan, their cards are exactly like those of other participants in the plan, so that only a technical person can determine that a client is actually financed by Multnomah County.

2. **Freedom of choice** of health plan.

   Each client is counselled about the various types of plans in an unbiased manner so an intelligent choice of a plan to meet his apparent needs, at a price he can afford to pay, can be made.

3. **Consumer cost participation.**

   The Project Health client shares in the cost of health cover- age on two levels.  One is based on ability to pay, and the other is based on the difference in costs between the commu- nity rate of the plan selected and the lowest cost plan.  In other words, the client that selects a more expensive health plan pays a proportionately higher monthly enrollment fee.

4. **Marketplace competition** stimulation.

   It was believed that if the various health plans were encour- aged to compete on the basis of the premium and the client enrollment fee, some cost containment could be achieved.  It was desired that the plans compete on the basis of their dif- ferent delivery systems cost, rather than the difference in risk or possible variation in utilization by the client.

5. **Cost containment** through prepayment.

   Project staff believed that HMOs had demonstrated at least some possibility for the prediction of a uniform cost over a period of time.  The prepaid health care plans administer the system.  Therefore, Project Health did not have to duplicate a costly system that already existed in the community.  This is a significant departure from government's traditional de- pendence on inflationary fee-for-service fee schedules and institutional cost reimbursement systems with their atten- dant large administrative bureaucracy.  Hopefully, in this

way, the high cost of the government's traditionally ineffective patch-work regulatory schemes could be avoided. Although there is no precise methodology of measuring the impact in Project Health's small laboratory, staff feel that
its point in cost containment has been proven.

6.    Health maintenance coverage.

Project Health's clients are enrolled for as lengthy periods
of coverage as possible, in order that their status of health
might be improved and their behavior modified from the traditional illness orientation through education and by utilization of the services of the system. Each client is locked into the health plan selected for at least 12 months, so that
the client cannot jump from one plan to another.

7.    Decategorization of government health care funding.

"Pooling" has been attempted in order to get government funds
into a program that may be allocated for the payment of a single service, a single disease entity, or a single categorical
client, and to use these funds to finance prepaid comprehensive health care for the eligible whole person. That is, dollars are put together to buy care for people. The Project
Health concept also results in a centralization of the administration of public health care financing and access, which reduces the costly duplication of bureaucratic overhead. This
centralization of administation and financing of health care
is one cost containment method that Project Health has demonstrated.

8.    Financial assistance to clients, not to health care providers.

Project Health subsidizes eligible clients and assists them
as consumers in utilizing health care coverage rather than
giving financial assistance to providers. Contracts with
plans and individual providers of all disciplines are set up
and staff assures, directs and monitors the access to this
health care coverage as an advocate of the client, rather than
of the provider. The purpose is to pay health care providers
in the mainstream for serving low income people in the same
way, with the same quality of care, as they service all other
people in the community. At the same time, these providers
are paid the same fees, or the same premiums, the community
as a whole pays for a like service.

9.    Consumer education and advocacy.

The Client Services Section is responsible for informing the
clients before enrollment, in order that they may better understand the available health plan options and make an informed
choice of the health plan they deem will best satisfy their
needs within their capacity to pay the enrollment fee. In
addition, this information helps the client utilize the bene-

fits of the health plan in a wiser and more appropriate manner than they otherwise would. There is follow-up with the client and the plans on an as needed basis to help them better utilize or break any of the barriers to access found in the health plans themselves.

10. Comprehensive benefits.

A benefit package that is comprehensive in nature provides a full range of medical benefits to the clients, including full hospitalization, outpatient office visits, prescriptions, physical examinations, and eye examinations. This is in direct contrast to the limited benefit packages offered through the illness-orientation of most government health programs.

Description of the Project in Terms of How It Operates, Its Funding and Its Clients

Figures 1 and 2 illustrate how Project Health operates as a "broker" for its clients and how its prepaid and episodic enrollment process functions. Appendices A and B describe the sources of funding for Project Health and how these funds were spent for years 1979-1980 and 1980-1981.

Summary--Project Health: Its Weaknesses and Strengths

1. Weaknesses

  - The size of the Project has been too small to constitute a good research data base. It has been difficult to test the instruments, e.g., have cost containment strategies held down rates or has success been due to aggressive negotiation activities and political power.

  - The medically needy (indigent) population has an apparent "illness" orientation or has, in fact, more indepth illness.

  - Limited resources have dictated turning away applicants toward the end of each fiscal year.

  - The local government built-in administrative restrictions have been difficult to work with.

  - The utilization patterns of the medically needy population were not well known and still are too variable to be actuarially ratable for risk assumption when Independent Practice Associations Prepaid Health Plans, Health Insurance Organizations and Group Practice Prepaid Health Plans are used as alternate options.

  - The County General Fund has not kept up with inflation and services continue to decrease.

2. Strengths

  - The medically needy in Multnomah County have received financ-

# Project Health
## The "Broker"

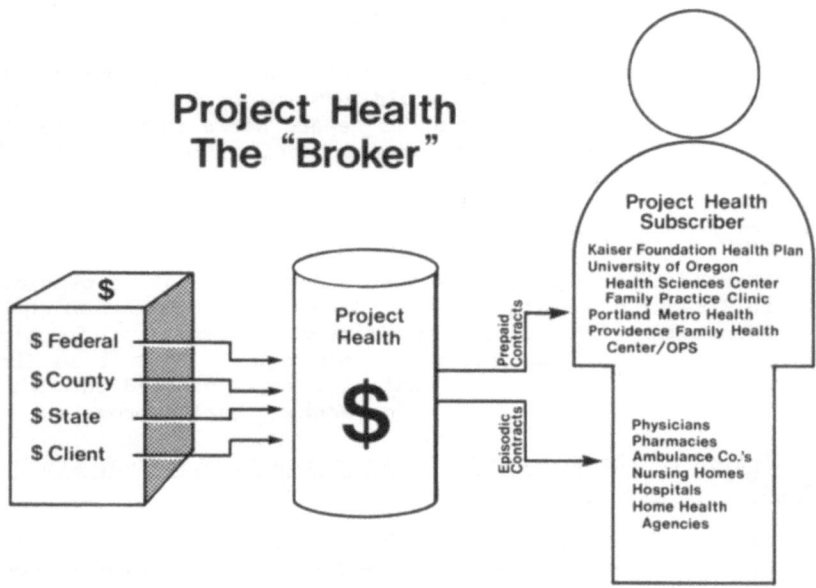

# Project Health: Prepaid and Episodic
## Enrollment Process

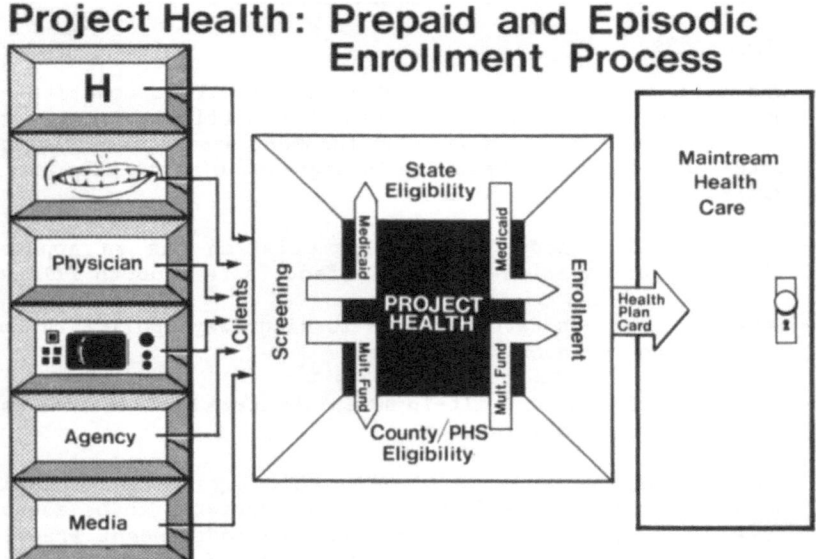

ing for the first time in history--an expanded Medicaid Program.

- Clients and providers are, for the most part, pleased with Project Health.

- Project Health's success and efforts encouraged the State Welfare Agency to contract with prepaid plans for care of the
Aid to Families with Dependent Children population--a new
experience.

- Unit costs of medical services were generally higher in the
Project Health episodic system than in the State Welfare Agency model, yet total per capita medical expenditures for the
medically needy are lower using the Project Health model than
for the State Welfare Agency model.  The major reason for the
apparent success of the Project Health "brokerage" model in
containing the costs of medical care appears to be the rates
negotitated with prepaid plans, which closely approximate community rates for individual enrollees in such plans.

- Low income residents have been enrolled in non-stigmatized
mainstream care.

- Project Health's concept has been nationally recognized as an
important cost containment strategy.

Appendix A

PROJECT HEALTH DOLLARS:   1979/80

WHERE THEY CAME FROM

| | | |
|---|---|---|
| Multnomah County | $4,549,826 | 48.2% |
| PHS 330 | 2,194,503 | 23.2% |
| Medicaid | 2,449,725 | 26.0% |
| Client Payments | 150,776 | 1.6% |
| Provider Refunds | 94,780 | 1.0% |
| Total | $9,439,610 | 100.0% |

AND WHERE THEY WENT

| | | |
|---|---|---|
| Services | $8,348,501 | 88.4% |
| Administration | 1,091,109 | 11.6% |
| Total | $9,439,610 | 100.0% |

APPENDIX B

PROJECT HEALTH DOLLARS:  1980/81

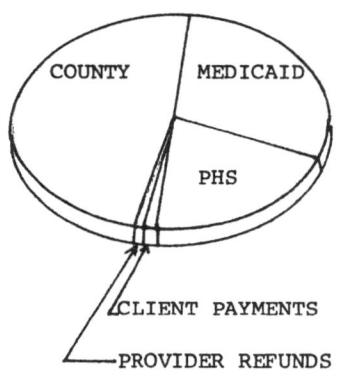

### WHERE THEY WILL COME FROM

| | | |
|---|---:|---:|
| Multnomah County | $4,178,226 | 46.4% |
| PHS 330 | 1,949,846 | 21.6% |
| Medicaid | 2,635,510 | 29.3% |
| Client Payments | 196,486 | 2.2% |
| Provider Refunds | 42,020 | .5% |
| Total | $9,002,088 | 100.0% |

### AND WHERE THEY WILL GO

| | | |
|---|---:|---:|
| Services | $7,574,542 | 84.1% |
| Research | 250,000 | 2.8% |
| Administration | 1,177,546 | 13.1% |
| Total | $9,002,088 | 100.0% |

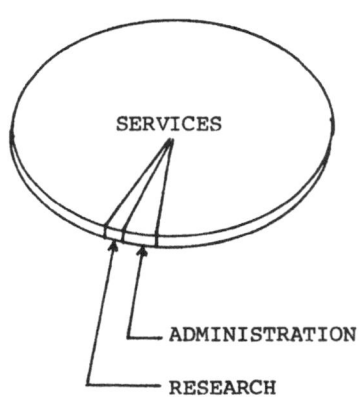

# RESPONSE
# Jesse H. Turner, Sr.

Multnomah County, Oregon, appears to be making a determined effort to control the costs and quality of its health care by purchasing primary health care under competitive contracts with primary care physicians. Perhaps, it should be emphasized that regardless of the success or failure of Project Health, it has made a meaningful contribution in the area of cost containment by focusing national and local attention on its efforts.

Its activities as a "broker" for prepaid health care are certainly beneficial to the poor who are usually ill-educated, and who, too often, fail to understand the terms and conditions of health agreements. To have experienced and knowledgeable personnel negotiating health care contracts on their behalf and supervising implementation thereof has to be pleasant reassurance for indigent persons.

Efforts by the Project toward non-stigmatizing mainstream health care for the indigent is, unquestionably, welcomed by low income recipients, who, too often, have to suffer indignities in receiving benefits because of their lack of political power.

Moreover, as a pioneer in alternative health care delivery service, Project Health generates grant awards and additional funds for the community as a demonstration project. Hopefully, this additional revenue will continue until many of the contentions of consumer-oriented-choice health plan adherents can be tried and evaluated. However, the potential for success of the project on a community-wide basis has been severely limited by limitation of its resources.

Even though Project Health is experiencing a degree of success in Multnomah County, Oregon--a county with seven alternative delivery systems, a somewhat homogenous population with about seven percent of its families below the poverty level, and a minority population of approximately five percent, including four percent black--one has to wonder how this experience would fare in the cities and communities across this country which have a large minority and/or indigent population.

Shelby County, Tennessee, with a population of approximately 750,000, 37 percent of whom are black and 21 percent of whom are below the poverty level, offers such a challenge. The county has only one alternative health care delivery system in operation with another scheduled to open shortly.

The Shelby County health care system appears to have more hospital resources per person and, apparently, uses these resources at a higher rate than Multnomah County. Some evidence of this disparity is shown by the following hospital data, supplied by Inter-Study, on the use of hospitals in Portland and Memphis, the major city in Shelby County. However, these data may require adjustments due to use of those hospital facilities by patients who reside outside the metropolitan areas.

|  | Portland | Shelby County |
|---|---|---|
| Beds/1000 pop. | 3.8 | 6.0 |
| Admissions/1000 pop. | 152 | 214 |
| Inpatient days/1000 pop. | 980 | 1705 |
| Length of Stay | 6.4 | 8.0 |

The Shelby County Commission is currently funding $19 million of a $26 million budget request by the Hospital Authority for the operation of the county hospital, approximately 80 percent of whose patients are black because the private hospitals have failed to assume their share of the services provided to indigent blacks.

Currently, there exists a controversy in Shelby County among the public hospital authority, the University of Tennessee Medical School and the County Commission as to the relationship of each in the operation of the hospital.

Racial segregation in housing in the county continues to increase as a result of continuing white flight and overt action by public officials to maintain that trend. The major private hospitals in the county are using their resources to perpetuate this trend by constructing new hospital facilities in the areas of white flight.

Moreover, the educational level of the black community remains below that of the white community; blighted housing conditions among blacks continue; and the income gap between blacks and whites is widening.

Given the above, it appears that neither the conditions or the climate are favorable for a successful and desired change in the health care delivery system of Shelby County.

To summarize, some of the obstacles to meaningful and immediate changes in this county are:

1.  Alternative health care systems are not available to offer competition to the existing system.

2.  The fact that blacks constitute such a large part of the indigent patient population lessens the pressure on the community to affect a change until it is shown that such change will reduce the health care budget.

3.  Continuing neighborhood segregation plus increasing hospital beds in locations of white flight will increase segregation in health care, thereby giving the community a better opportunity to ignore the health of the black community.

4.  The failure of the private hospitals to accept their share of black indigent patients while, on the other hand, accepting and assimilating white indigent patients with their other patients further entrenches segregation and abets stigmatization of delivery of health care to the black population.

5.  The low educational level of the indigent patients will require a longer and more expensive educational program to sell any proposed change.

In this country, the private sector has a poor record of providing equitable services for blacks. This results in almost continuous clamor by this segment of our community for federal regulations to attain equity. Regretfully, the health care industry's record is no better than that of the nation as a whole.

Thus, one can anticipate vigorous opposition by blacks to any plan which tends to reduce governmental regulation or close public hospitals which, regardless of their faults, have provided blacks with whatever health care they have received.

Finally, the black community is witnessing attempts in this country today to dismantle the public school system and to institute a voucher system for education primarily to aid and abet those private, segregated schools which have sprung up to provide an outlet for those whites who have deserted public schools to avoid desegregation. With such a long history of benign neglect no one then can expect blacks to support a voucher system for health care which acceptance would probably be used by proponents of racial segregation as a support for continued segregation of education. Despite the benefits contained in the proposals advocated by Dr. Enthoven in his new book Health Plan it appears unlikely that any material change will be made in the delivery of health care in this country in the near future until and unless there is strong outside pressure.

# V
# THE MINNEAPOLIS-ST. PAUL EXPERIENCE
## Glenn D. Nelson

Following is a description of the current Twin Cities health care marketplace, with special reference to the presence of alternate delivery systems, and speculation as to the future health care system which may evolve in the Twin Cities. Hopefully, this discussion will provide insights which will influence the development of new approaches in other parts of the country.

It has been said that the Twin Cities are unique in their health care system and thus may not represent an appropriate model for replication. Several points must be offered in this regard:

1. To a large degree, the Twin Cities evolved into their current unique state from a more traditional form.

2. Virtually any health care marketplace in the nation could be considered unique in its particular demographic, medical and social situations.

3. The purpose of examining the Twin Cities experience is to gain perspectives and specific facts, not to suggest wholesale replication of the system.

Therefore, the review of the Twin Cities experience will be done in such a fashion as to identify features of importance in developing health care systems to meet the major health systems challenges of the future: cost, quality and access.

It is suggested that a thoughtful review of the system may result in an emphasis on new approaches to health care, rather than mere modifications to the existing system.

The Minneapolis/St. Paul metropolitan area has a current population of 2,000,000, with only a ten percent growth predicted by 1990. The following tables describe some of the important parameters of the Twin Cities health systems today.

Table 1:  HOSPITAL DATA

| Hospital Data (Community Hospitals) | Minneapolis/St. Paul | All SMSAs | InterStudy Adequacy Levels* |
|---|---|---|---|
| # of hospitals | 39 | | |
| # of beds | 11,117 | | |
| Beds/1000 pop. | 5.4 | 4.5 | 3.0 max. |
| Hospital employees/ 1000 pop. | 14.7 | 13.3 | 9 max. |
| Admissions/1000 pop. | 169 | 161 | 130 max. |
| Inpatient days/1000 pop. | 1398 | 1256 | 800 max. |
| Occupancy rate | 71.1% | 76.0% | 85.0% min. |
| Length of stay | 8.3 | 7.8 | |
| Surgeries/1000 | 87.2 | 85.5 | |
| Expenses inpatient day | $232.85 | $240.81 | |
| Expenses/capita | $325.46 | $302.54 | |

Table 2:  PHYSICIAN DATA

| Physician Data (Non-Federal) | Minneapolis/St. Paul | All SMSAs | Total U.S. |
|---|---|---|---|
| Active Physicians (MDs) | 3,728 | 272,818 | 315,745 |
| Physicians/1000 | 1.8 | 1.75 | 1.48 |
| % General Practice | 14.4% | 11.3% | 14.3% |
| % Medical Specialities | 17.6% | 19.6% | 19.0% |
| % Surgical Specialities | 18.5% | 23.0% | 23.2% |
| % Other Specialities | 15.9% | 17.1% | 16.7% |
| % Hospital Based | 33.7% | 29.0% | 26.8% |
| % of MDs in Residency | 13.5% | 19.5% | 17.3% |

In 1971, prepaid health care was a very small factor in the Twin
Cities, with 42,000 members cared for by the Group Health Plan
formed as a cooperative in 1956. However, in the late 1960s and
early 1970s, Paul Ellwood, citizens groups, business task forces
and health providers actively considered the issues of prepaid
health care. It was in that climate that a multi-specialty group
practice, the St. Louis Park Medical Center (Center) sponsored a
second health maintenance organization (HMO). As a result, a new
form of health care competition arose in the Twin Cities. In 1972,
when the Center founded its HMO, the MedCenter Health Plan, it had
only 69 physicians providing service at one location.

Today, the Center is a multi-specialty group practice with a staff
of 130 physicians and 678 support personnel. Care is provided at
seven outpatient facilities. The Center does not own or control
any hospital facilities. Many diagnostic and surgical services
which might ordinarily be associated with hospital care are provided in an outpatient setting. Approximately 33 percent of the
Center's activities is prepaid, while 65 percent is still traditional fee-for-service activities. The group's growth has been at-
tributed to a number of factors, but clearly the addition of a prepaid option brought many new patients to the Center and was probably
responsible for about 40 percent of the new growth since 1972. It
also brought increased visibility to the group and probably additional fee-for-service activities. Clearly the most significant
result was the subsequent development in 1976 of the Physicians
Health Plan formed by the County Medical Society. This plan involved most of the Society's membership who saw the need to respond
to the competition of the three existing HMOs.

Certain aspects of the Center's entry into the HMO market in the
Twin Cities should be emphasized. It appears that integrated multi-
group practices, like the Center, use fewer hospital bed days in-
herently in providing health care to similar patient populations
than is the usual community average. When the Center entered prepayment, it was using 400 bed days per 1000 people, whereas the community average was between 800 and 900 beds. As a result, early
financial viability was assured. The group's efficient use of the
total health dollar was unmasked by the prepayment mechanism. It
should be noted that the arrival of prepayment at the Center did
not have the expected adverse effect on its primary hospitals, because efficient utilization already existed. The Center did not
need to reduce hospital utilization to achieve its actuarial
goals.

Several additional points should be made in reference to the multi-
specialty group practice in terms of its adaptability for prepayment. Multi-specialty group practices tend to share records, which
results in the sharing of diagnostic information, and a reduction
in both repetition within the system and lost information. This
may expedite outcome in a cost-effective fashion. Also, these group
practices have the physical plants and financial strength to develop
the capacity for ambulatory diagnostic and therapeutic approaches
which is clearly an advantage as they enter prepayment.

Two of the most frequent challenges about the prepayment mechanism
are that it will lead to skimming and poor quality care. In the St.

Louis Park setting, improved quality assurance mechanisms have been instituted that provide some remarkable insights about medical outcome.  In fact, the Center's attempts to improve quality have been greatly enhanced by the existence of the prepayment mechanism. Patients are followed to outcome and mechanisms have been instituted to determine patients' understanding of their role  in their health care.  It has been observed that patient satisfaction tends to lead to greater compliance and better outcomes.  Obviously, patient satisfaction is critical in an organization that is selling prepaid health care, and there is a dual motive for achieving this satisfaction--enrollment and medical outcome.

Another effect apparent in the community when the Center began offering prepayment was that patients began transferring care from their previous physicians because of the new financing mechanism. The response of other health care providers to the patient movement resulted in a cascade of new HMOs over the ensuing four years.

| | |
|---|---|
| Coordinated Health Care | 1973 |
| SHARE | 1973 |
| Nicollet Eitel | 1973 |
| HMO Minnesota | 1974 |
| Physicians Health Plan | 1976 |

In summary, multi-specialty group practices have some inherent features that facilitate transition to the prepayment mechanism:

1.    Less reliance on the hospital and hospitalization of patients to administer care.

2.    Less duplication of therapeutic and diagnostic procedures because of the integration of the health care providers and their record system.

3.    Patient transfer from existing physicians is a strong motivator for competitive responses in developing alternative delivery systems.

4.    High quality health care could be less expensive when outcome analysis is the determinant.

Current State

The following graph reflects the increase in enrollment in Twin Cities HMOs from 1971 to 1979.  The enrollment rate has been accelerating through 1980.  (Figure 1).  The Twin Cities has slightly more than 2,000,000 people in its ten-county Minneapolis/St. Paul metropolitan area at this time.  The growth rate is less than one percent a year.  The area includes a large academic medical center

and is a regional medical care area, providing tertiary care to
people living outside the cities (approximately 18 percent of all
metropolitan area patients are non-residents). It is felt that
the metropolitan area probably has an excess number of hospital
beds and physicians even considering the fact that a significant
number of patients come from outside the metropolitan area. The
ability of the alternate delivery systems to grow and prosper may
have been, in fact, related to the ease of acquiring physician
staffing and hospital beds in the marketplace.

TWIN CITIES HMO ENROLLMENT/1000 People

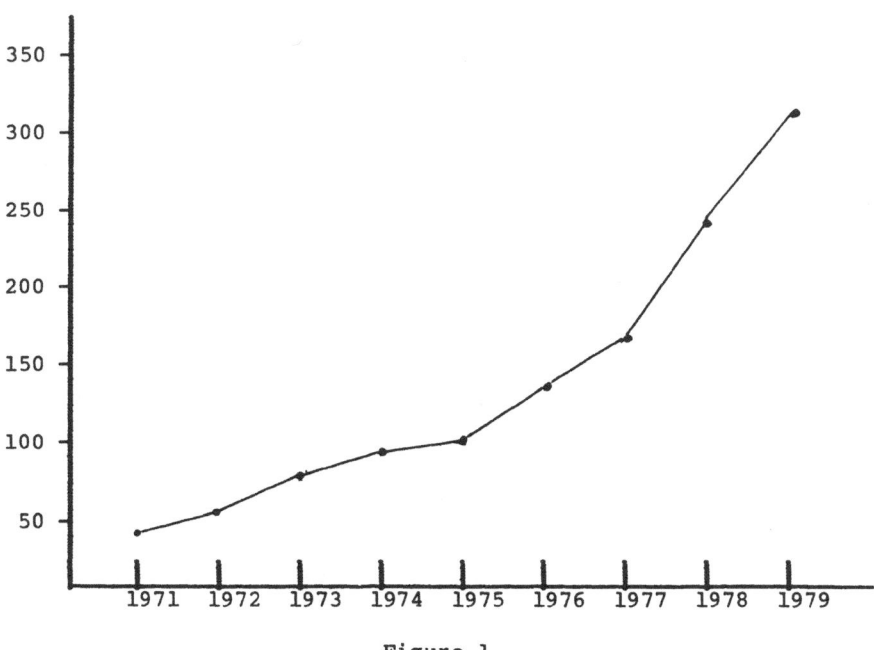

Figure 1

The prepaid activities have had a dramatic impact, aside from the
new enrollee annual component growth at 30 percent. At this time,
approximtely 75-80 percent of all physicians in the metropolitan
area are involved in one or more of the HMOs. The physicians or
their sponsoring groups are becoming proactive in attempting to
control their costs through more appropriate utilization of health
resources. Employers have begun to recognize the substantial savings that have been achieved in some instances, and they are actively supporting the prepayment options.

Health care costs in the Twin Cities are down, as compared to the national average. Hospital bed days per 1000 in the past two years
have declined 4.5 percent, versus one percent nationally. In 1979,

the consumer price index (CPI) medical care component in Minneapolis rose 6.8 percent versus 9.9 percent for all cities.  This is
particularly significant in view of the fact that overall CPI in
Minneapolis went up 11.9 percent versus 11.5 percent for other
U.S. cities.

The illustrations demonstrating admissions per 1000 people and
patient bed days per 1000 people in Minneapolis/St. Paul versus
U.S. averages are striking.  It is interesting to note that admission rates and the bed days per 1000 rate are both above U.S.
averages, which in part reflects in-migration to the metropolitan
area for health care.  More important, is the fact that both these
parameters are clearly declining at the same time the U.S. averages are flat.  (Figures 2 and 3).

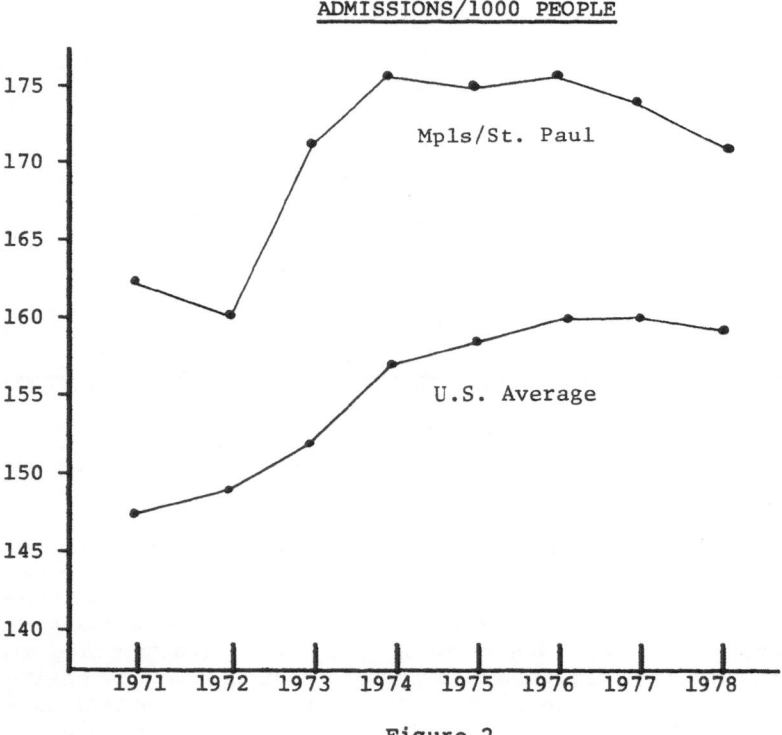

ADMISSIONS/1000 PEOPLE

Mpls/St. Paul

U.S. Average

Figure 2

PATIENT DAYS/1000 PEOPLE

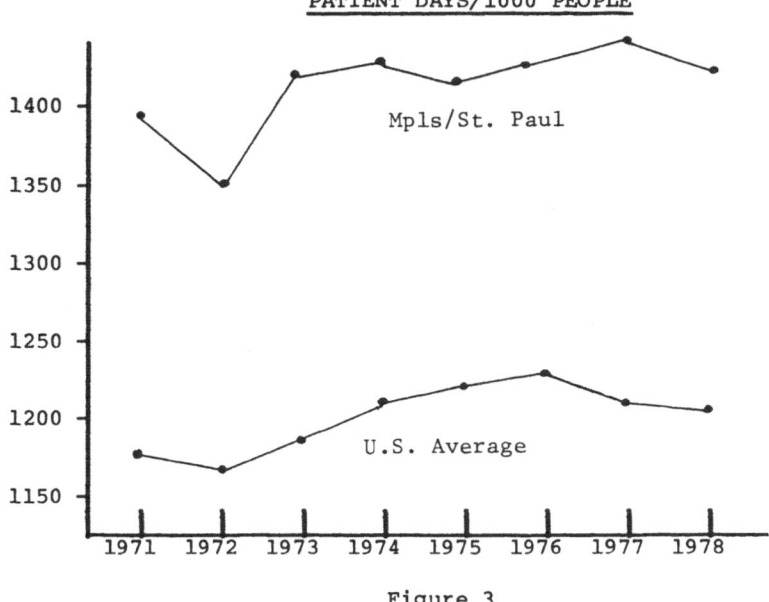

Figure 3

A Medicare demonstration project is being developed but very few Medicare patients are currently cared for by the HMOs in Minneapolis/St. Paul, and yet the Medicare costs are showing a relative decline in the area.  It is presumed that there is some spillover effect as regards the physicians' attitudes about utilization (particularly in the hospital).

It could be argued that the decline in hospital utilization is related to factors other than competition.  Utilization review programs instituted by agencies and hospitals may have played a role.  However, the compelling fact is that the Twin Cities are different from the national trends in its reduction of hospital admissions and it is most likely that the drop in admissions among the non-HMO population is a spillover effect from the newly perceived standards resulting from HMO utilization efforts.

The consumer of health care is benefiting from the movement in several ways.  There are many new sites of access in the neighborhoods and shopping areas convenient to patients, rather than in physician office buildings adjacent to existing hospitals.  Health professionals are making themselves available on a regular basis in the evenings and at other non-traditional hours.  Ambulatory surgery and outpatient care is promoted, saving the patients time and anxiety.  Finally, there is new emphasis on health education, preventive medicine and "wellness."  People of the community are learning more about what is being offered by various physician groups and presumably are becoming better buyers of care.

The Future

Most observers of the Twin Cities marketplace believe that prepayment will continue to involve an ever-larger portion of the population and could reach 50 percent of the population by 1985. Such growth will likely produce some consolidation or merger of the provider elements of the health care system. Certainly, hospital merger or realignment may be precipitated in such an environment, and hospitals may take a more proactivist position in responding to the various alternative health delivery systems in an effort to stabilize their activities. Entities removed from the current health care system, or peripheral to it, may begin to view the opportunities as an avenue for entrepreneurial involvement because of the large dollars involved. The enlarging physician surplus will certainly allow provider entities an unrestricted work force. Advancing technology in the diagnostic and information systems areas will be so sophisticated as to require sophisticated organizations to maximize the potential. Medical care will move from its infancy in management utilization. Finally, the emphasis on wellness will result in new initiatives for preventive medicine and self care.

# RESPONSE
# Frank A. Sloan

Unlike the Twin Cities, the Mid-South is underpopulated with alternative delivery systems. It is important to understand why there is a shortage and what can be done to bring about a more thorough implementation of new systems within the region.

I discuss these issues as an economist. The notion of competition is not one that has to lead only to cost control; it can also lead to quality assurance. The proponents of competition want to make a deliberate choice about both payment and quality.

Not too long ago some economists said it did not matter what share of the gross national product (GNP) was devoted to health. If people wanted good health care then there may be nothing wrong with a large share of the GNP going for these services. However, although health care does have a lot to offer, so do many other sectors of the economy. Americans are faced with cost and productivity pressures. The era of cost containment is here, and it is becoming a question of what "weapon" we are going to choose to control health care costs. Are we going to choose a regulatory system, or one that incorporates at least some market-oriented principles? Even if nothing is done, costs will increase during the 1980s due to technological change, an increasing supply of physicians, changes in the demographic mix of the population, and an increasingly aged population. The issue, in making the comparisons between needs competing with health care, is what kind of system best serves our society's purposes.

Undoubtedly, regulation has often not worked. It has proved to be inequitable; it has not recognized the diversity of the population it serves; and it has not provided for coordination among regulatory agencies. One type of regulatory program that does seem to have worked in terms of cost containment is the prospective reimbursement system for hospitals. A number of studies suggest this type of program has limited costs, but there may be unfortunate side effects such as the closing of hospitals in indigent areas.

There is a base of evidence on regulation, but very limited information on competitive strategies. There are case studies which provide useful clues, but they are only clues as to what would happen if the United States went from a system of a few cities with 20 percent of their population participating in alternative delivery systems, to a system in which there was a nationwide participation of much more than 20 percent.

In the absence of very complete knowledge, we should proceed incrementally.  We are not ready for a full-fledged program, but need demonstration programs, particularly in cities with substantial indigent populations and in rural areas.  Hopefully these demonstration programs will include many different types of alternative delivery systems, and not just evaluate large-scale prepaid group practices.

The demonstration programs do not have to be operated as scientific experiments with tests and controls.  Rather there should be doing and then eye-balling results to get a feel for the problems.  There will be tremendous political opposition to new health care models until there is a much more national, widespread experience to show that new models can work in rural counties, as well as in large metropolitan counties, such as Shelby County in Tennessee.

The health care system is extremely complex and involves numerous parties.  Certainly, the consumer must be considered, although one wonders why the consumer up to now has not been more cost conscious.  There must be concern for special groups of consumers with special needs such as the indigent.

Employers have a major role in the development of alternative delivery systems, although this group also has not been very cost conscious in the past.  Unions also have a role.  Traditionally unions have not been strong supporters of alternative delivery systems.  Methods for involving them in this process need to be developed.

Another important party is the regulators.  There have been fears in some areas that regulators might be an impediment to the development of alternative delivery systems.  For example, certificate-of-need requirements may make it more difficult for hospitals with alternative delivery affiliations to come on line.

Still another party is the "trust buster."  What are the policies of the U.S. Justice Department, the Federal Trade Commission, and state attorney generals going to be toward alternative delivery systems?  Will some of these systems, such as independent practice associations, be viewed as anti-competitive from an anti-trust standpoint?

There is the individual physician.  What happens when 50 percent instead of five percent of the population is being served by alternative delivery systems?  Also important is the posture of organized medicine, which years ago was opposed to a number of these alternative delivery systems, but in recent years has become much more supportive, although they are still cautious.

Another group to consider is the health professional other than the physician.  What role will be played under these competitive models by nurse practitioners, physician's assistants, etc.? Still another party is the academic health center which presents a definite cost problem with respect to competitive strategies.

Looking at these alternative systems and asking why they have not been more widely implemented, it is clear that all these parties, which have sometimes competing and sometimes consistent interests, are one reason. The challenge before the health professions and others in the health industry is to bring all of the parties together to implement new delivery systems and contain cost.

# VI
# THE BUSINESS PERSPECTIVE
# OF HEALTH
## Henry E. Simmons

As a prelude to this presentation, it is important to understand the economic conditions that are likely to prevail for the health care system and industry in the 1980s. Most analysts have concluded that the decade is destined to be unusually troubled and uncertain. They predict continued serious inflation, slowing of productivity gain, slow real economic growth, perhaps the slowest since World War II, decreased purchasing power for individual consumers, and probably a decrease in the average standard of living. Clearly these predicted conditions will have a profound effect on the nation's industries and health care system.

With the United States facing severe continued inflation and a troubled economy, the problem of massive and rapidly rising health care costs will be either the major or one of the major social issues of the 80s. It is not hard to understand why. Per capita health costs have doubled in the past decade. With a faltering economy and slowing productivity gains, these costs are likely to prove intolerable for both government and society. The result will be increasingly fierce competition among health care providers because (1) ever increasing cost mainfests itself in system shrinkage and reorganization as only those who are competitive will survive, and (2) the big buyers, government and industry, are convinced that perhaps one third or more of the health care they pay for does not serve their, or their constituents, best interest.

Given the total resource constraints buyers now face, industry leaders feel that they can no longer sit by and let the health care system operate as it has in the past, consuming more and more of their available resources in what I view as a wasteful fashion. These buyers will force change, and they will begin to deal preferentially with those providers who can provide quality services efficiently and economically.

Government and industry have become convinced that the status quo in medical care is unacceptable and that changes must come because they have come to accept the following as facts. One, health care costs have increased more than three fold in the past decade, and are rising at rates substantially higher than the rate of general inflation.

Two, output of the health care system, in terms of benefits to employees and society, is nowhere near commensurate with the resources expended. Although the United States is already operating the most expensive health care system in the world, no end is in sight for increasing costs. In fact, the nation is faced with a bill of $785 billion by 1990 if present trends continue.

Three, much of the medical care delivered has no proven benefit. There is a substantial body of evidence that ever higher costs are not necessarily equated with higher quality care, or better health outcomes. In fact, evidence is accumulating that in many instances, the exact opposite is true. Real quality care will be achieved by doing less than what is currently being done and to fewer patients.

Four, within broad ranges, there appears to be no significant correlation between, on the one hand, the level of health of the population served and, on the other hand, the number and level of training of physicians available, the amount spent for health care, the setting in which care is rendered or the number of hospital beds.

A recent article in the New England Journal of Medicine by Walter McNerney, President of Blue Cross, characterized this belief. Basically he concluded that only ten percent of all the premature deaths in this country can be affected by the traditional health care system. The rest lies outside that domain, and will be affected by behavioral and environmental changes which traditional medical care cannot reach.

Industry looking at its own utilization statistics is finding marked regional and often inter- and intra-institutional variations in hospital utilization rates and treatment patterns for their employees, variations not explainable on the basis of disease or medical care. In addition, in some areas of the country, employees are using one half to one third as many hospital beds as in other areas, without any adverse effects to the population served.

The steel industry is an example. In one geographical area, employees had a patient utilization rate of 1900 per 1000, almost five times the rate of efficient health maintenance organizations (HMO). Industry officials took this information to the medical society. As a result, the society is sending a bulletin to its members which begins:

> "After years of concern and months of preparation, we would like to send you, fellow physicians, the following note:
>
>> As noted, national health care costs have risen strikingly in recent years. Also the local business community has insisted that health

care costs are higher in our county than in
many other areas of our country. Comparative
data acquired from Blue Cross and from national corporations with operations here, corro-
borate the existence of a particularly severe
cost problem in our community. An analysis of
these data indicate that the increased cost
in our area is due, in large part, to an unusually high number of hospital admissions for
our population. Excessive use of the hospital
may result from our practice habits and could
be influenced by the presence of excessive
hospital beds and prevailing mechanisms of
reimbursement. While each of us may not totally agree with the conclusions for proposed
actions of these groups (industry) we ignore
them at our peril."

The bulletin continues with a description of an extensive program
of utilization review and other steps physicians should take to
control health care costs.

Memphis statistics are particularly interesting. Memphis' days
per 1000 are 1700; the U.S. average is 1200. Admissions per 1000
are 214; the U.S. average is 162. Industry knows that quality care
is being delivered to millions of Americans today with less than
half and in some instances one quarter of those kinds of rates.
They also know that with, or even without, alternative delivery
systems, in some communities bed utilization rates have been decreased by one half to one third with no adverse effect to the population and with a freeing up of resources for use in areas of equal
or greater need.

These are the facts that industry has become convinced characterize
the present health care system. Who is pushing these facts? It is
not just a bunch of wild-eyed idealistic liberals pushing for national health insurance. These facts are being laid out by some
of the nations most respected medical experts from medical centers
across the country. They are being presented to industry and are
being backed by credible scientific studies. The United States
Chamber of Commerce is increasingly taking this information to its
members and pointing out that the status quo cannot continue. Concern about the rising total cost of health care coupled with the
realization that much of the health care delivered today is unnecessary or inefficiently provided, will drive reform in the system
for it is now clear that quality health care will be delivered only
when attention is paid to the cost of that care.

Why must industry act? Because what started out as truly a fringe
benefit, a cost which could always be passed on to the purchasers
of industry products, has come to constitute, next to energy, the
biggest and most rapidly growing uncontrollable cost of doing business, actually threatening the profitability of some industries,

which have seen a 250 percent increase in their medical benefit costs in just four years.  The steel industry found that in 1978 its health benefit costs represented 45 percent of its total profits.  Even in years when the economy was healthy, industry could not remain profitable with this kind of an uncontrolled cost escalation.  Now many major industries are in trouble--automobile, steel, rubber.  Corporate profits decreased a record $19 billion recently.  Not long ago, the world's largest corporation, General Motors, reported that its aging plants were going to need billions of dollars for modernization.  The same story exists in the steel industry.  The reindustrialization of America  will require profits and one of the biggest recent drains on profits in many industries is medical benefit costs.  The most frightening thing to industry is that it sees no end in sight in the health care cost escalation spiral.  This realization makes industry determined to begin to use its billions of dollars of purchasing power to force change. Industry will not tolerate, and can no longer afford the status quo.

Industry is being joined in this concern by a new ally, unions, as unions begin to see that in this area their interests coalesce with industry.  Unions see that health care costs appear to be a bottomless pit; the health care system seems able to absorb every dollar allocated to it.

Unions see that if increasingly limited corporate profits are spent for health care benefits, less and less money is left on the bargaining table to pay for wage increases.  Therefore, industry and unions are beginning a dialogue which consists of the following: we are both wasting a great deal of money in the health care system; why not begin to work together to control that amount because without sacrificing quality, very substantial amounts of dollars can be freed for other important purposes.

This dialogue is having results.  In the last steel industry negotiations, the United Steel Workers of America agreed to a medical necessity provision, utilization review, second opinion surgery, increased deductibles, home health care benefits, and modifications in the benefit package to encourage out-of-hospital care.

The end result of the liaison between industry and unions will be cuts in the use of medical resources, particuarly hospital inpatient care.  It is reasonable to assume that the next step industry and unions take will be to preferentially bargain with and utilize efficient providers and insurers and place some type of penalty on employees who insist on utilizing unnecessarily expensive or inefficient providers.  In addition, where they do not find the system responsive to their needs, industry and unions may in some instances actually develop, create and operate their own delivery system. Industry dollars are large enough for them to do this, and the physician manpower glut makes such a unique approach feasible.

In my judgement, industries will increasingly be shopping for an approach which makes optimal use of their benefit dollars to favorably effect the health and the productivity of their employees, their families and retirees.  They are convinced this will not be accomplished through greater use of expensive medical specialists or tertiary care centers alone.  In fact, they now feel even heavier investment in traditional medical care will have very little ultimate payoff for their employees.  They will look for organized and efficient systems that can deliver care predominantly on an ambulatory care basis, heavily oriented to primary care, with the use of paraprofessionals, and with the capability of offering disease prevention and health education services.

The current health care system is beginning to change in response to these pressures.  Bed growth has slowed.  Ambulatory care has grown rapidly.  The number of hospitals has decreased, 200 fewer than several years ago.  Bankruptcies are occurring and are no longer automatically viewed as intolerable.  Finally, hospital mergers and consortia development are increasing in an attempt to achieve economies and control markets.

The corporate practice of medicine is a growing phenomenon as physicians band together to compete.  There already are, and soon will be more, instances of groups of physicians bargaining with hospitals for a preferential per diem rate for their patients.  The predictions are now that HMOs alone will probably capture almost 23 million Americans by the end of the decade.

The future of academic health centers in this changing system could be very bright.  Who else can provide the trained personnel to work as a team, the models for the delivery system and the quality of care to achieve needed changes?  The times provide a chance for leadership and involvement in change by academic health centers as well as the private practice of medicine.  For those willing to be responsive, opportunities are virtually limitless.

The times they are a changing, as they must.  Industry actions will continue to force change in the 80s.  In my judgement, this will lead to the development of a better, more responsive health care system, hopefully with a minimum of government intervention.  Ultimately, such a system is in the best interest not only of society, but of those who work in the system.

# VII
# NATIONAL HEALTH POLICY
# FOR THE 1980s
## Walter J. McClure

There is both good news and bad news as to national health policy for the 1980s. I will start with the bad news.

The medical care system of this country, although it helps many people, is in very serious trouble. Before that trouble can be resolved, the system must take some serious medicine. Some will believe that the cure may be worse than the disease.

There are caveats to this presentation. The first is, "It's always different in the South." But, since what is done in Washington does have some effect here, I will speak from a national perspective and what I say can be adjusted to Memphis and its environment.

The second caveat is a little more serious. There are problems with the medical care system. However, we must remind ourselves of the system's strengths. I would simply say that were I to be unfortunate enough to become ill, I would prefer to have my medical care in this country, than in any other, provided that I was well covered.

The third caveat is that we need to avoid the blame game. I have noticed a tendency in this country to find the guys with the black hats. People point fingers at the doctors who then point fingers at the government, and so on down the line. I do not think any one group is responsible for the problems; but regardless of who is responsible, everyone will have to live with the solutions. So although you may not be responsible for the problems, if you abdicate from working on the solutions, you have no one to blame but yourself for the final solutions reached.

The 1980s will be a decade of serious change in health care. I say that for one reason--money! The goals the medical care system wants to accomplish--adequate care and adequate coverage for everyone--are being delayed because of their high price tag. Even without reaching these accomplishments, medical care costs are eating Americans out of house and home. Those on the provider side of medical care must realize that those on the paying side, business and government, cannot take the cost anymore. Thus, business and government are going to have to make changes and will do so with or without provider support. It would be a tragedy if medicine were simply to hide its head in the sand and say, "We don't want any of this," because there is going to be change. Cost will force it because this country cannot have the cost of its third largest industry escalating chronically at half again the rate of the rest of the economy.

While President, Jimmy Carter decided one week to balance the budget. A week later he decided that was politically difficult, but during that one week the major item he could not get a handle on was the cost of Medicare and Medicaid. There was no way to control it, so the government decided it would save $1 million simply by refusing to pay its bills for six months. This was a serious policy suggestion of which those in the hospital industry should take note.

There are two important points about health care during the 1980s. One, there will be changes as this is the decade for recognizing finite limits in medical care. And two, the changes needed to have a cost-effective medical care system are not trivial. They are very serious and substantial.

If there is anything that I have seen in the decade of the 70s, it is a failure to appreciate this point. Following is an indication of just how serious the problem is. A cost-effective medical care system—a system that delivers high quality medical care in an efficient and cost conscious way—would require retiring at least 20 percent of the hospital capacity in this country. How do I know that? Because there are extremely reputable and prestigious institutions that achieve that kind of performance right now. I do not believe in moth-balling hospitals; that is not what should be done. The point is that this problem will not be solved by expressions of good will, by minor private sector actions, or by dinky public regulations. The voluntary effort, an effort by medicine and hospitals to collaborate in an organized manner to reduce hospital costs, is a sincere and well-intentioned plan, but I believe it is misguided because a voluntary effort cannot ultimately achieve what must be done. Can you imagine the Baptist Hospital in Memphis complacently letting their hospital go over the hill, while the Methodist did well? We are talking about coming to terms. In the automobile industry you can see what coming to terms with finite limits and efficiency has done. The defense industry's coming to terms may have gone too far. The Defense Department at one time consumed ten percent of the gross national product (GNP) of this country. In the same period that the cost of medical care rose from five to almost ten percent of GNP, defense costs fell from ten to five percent of GNP. The drop was not accidental. Resources are finite. If you overspend on one thing, you must spend less on something else.

Before a solution to this problem is prescribed, its diagnosis must be better understood. Cost is not the cause, it is a symptom.

The maldistribution of physicians is not a cause, it is a symptom. Excess hospital capacity is not a cause, it is a symptom. Our ability or inability to cover low income people adequately without aggravating inflation is not a cause, it is a symptom. These are all symptoms of a deeper underlying malady—the absence of effective market forces in the delivery of medical care. Most people hate to hear "Economics I" mentioned in the same breath with medical care. However, discussing economics along with medical care in no way detracts from the compassionate and caring aspects of medical care. By market failure or absence of effective market forces, I mean the incentives of the present system all penalize cost-effective behavior on the part of patients, physicians and hospitals. The more costly and elaborate the care rendered by a physician or hospital, the more revenue that is generated. Efficiency generates less revenue.

Adam Smith and his successors laid down certain conditions that a market must meet if competition is to serve the public interest. First, fair market conditions are needed or the market will fail. The health care industry lacks these conditions and must establish them. Second, if there are no competitors, there will not be a good market. Health care plans, health maintenance organizations, alliances, Safeco plans, and preferred physician arrangements are needed as competitive alternatives to the traditional fee-for-service system. It is not that we want to do away with traditional providers, it is merely that we want to give them serious competitors so that health competition on price as well as service factors will develop. Those in business and in government need to purchase services from these competitors in a fair way and not pay more toward one than another. If business and government do not buy right, effective market conditions will not exist and the benefits of competitive systems will not occur. Buying right and competiton must go hand in hand.

Two things can be done about these faulty incentives or market failures: (1) restructure the private medical care system to make competition work, or (2) use regulatory forces as a substitute for the missing market forces. The debate is often phrased as "competition versus regulation," but that is not accurate. There is enormous competition in the present medical care system but it is cost generating rather than cost saving because the system is in market failure. Therefore, what we are talking about is restructuring or reforming the market versus direct economic regulation where bureaucrats decide prices, practice criteria, manpower distribution and facility need.

This is the choice for the decade of the 80s—market reform or direct economic regulation. I cannot predict what will happen. I simply ask, which do you want to emphasize. Because if those in the private sector think that there has been enough government intervention in this economy, and that it is appropriate to try and reduce that level of intervention, then they will have to take the initiative to make effective competition happen. It will not happen by accident. If those in the private sector do nothing, government will proceed without them, and government on its own tends to come up with regulatory solutions.

The more market forces established in the private system the more likely it becomes that the system will perform well, and the less likely that regulation will be needed. Conversely, the less market forces the private sector establishes, the more problematic it becomes, in my judgment, that the system will perform well. Thus, if there are no market forces, stronger regulations will be needed and the medical care system will become a public utility.

Admittedly, public utilities are not all bad. Their benefits show up reasonably soon, whereas their problems take ten to twenty years to appear. These problems tend to lie in rigidity and red tape, in the stifling of innovation, in inefficiency and in a certain non-responsiveness to consumers. There is some indication that competition tends to do much better on these fronts. So I am simply going to advocate that competition be given a credible shot. If it does not work after five to ten years, the Canadian public utility solution can be implemented, because then there will be no other choice. On the other hand, if the public utility route is tried first and it fails, it will be very difficult to revert to competition.

One should not be misled by the fact that there is a new conservative administration in Washington. Many feel this administration will be pro-competition, but that is not known for sure. It may be pro-status quo, and the status quo is in market failure. If everyone goes to sleep because there is a conservative administration, the precious lead time that currently exists to get competition up and going will evaporate. Then when the government finally is in crisis because of rising Medicare and Medicaid costs, and someone is in charge who decides to balance the budget for longer than one week, there will be no choice but to regulate the health care industry because that will be the only choice available.

Very hard work and the confidence to ride through the problems until the competitive models catch hold are needed for the changes to succeed. The good news is it can be done, if, but only if, the private sector seizes the initiative and works flat out, starting now.

# VIII
# THE AMERICAN WAY OF MEDICAL CARE 1980-1990
## Paul M. Ellwood

The opportunity to discuss the delivery of health care in 1990 is an enviable assignment, because I am convinced the best way to shape the future is to predict the future, especially if you are willing to hedge by trying to make it happen.

I believe that a critical discontinuity is developing in the historical course of the American way of medical care. The momentum has shifted from a piecemeal, non-price competitive system towards a health system shaped by overt competition. In fact, many key decisions have been made and the crucial organizational models are in place to further the competitive movement. New public and private policies could slow or accelerate the process of change, but I doubt that any policy is likely to stop the movement toward a more classically competitive medical marketplace.

I will discuss four topics relating to competition in the delivery of health care.

1.  The shape of the new medical marketplace.

2.  The pace of change.

3.  Forecaster's clues. What evidence is there that health history will not repeat itself?

4.  The unfinished business; the fate of hospitals and academic medical centers is too uncertain to call.


The Shape Of The New Medical Marketplace

The shape of the new medical marketplace, described in detail by previous speakers, basically requires: (1) fair market choice for consumers, and (2) sets of providers competing with each other on price and services.  In a community like Memphis, for example, effective competition will exist when at least 75 percent of the physicians are aligned with price competitive arrangements, likely to take either of two forms:  (1) a model similar to a health maintenance organization (HMO), or (2) what has been labeled as "preferred provider organizations" (PPO).

PPOs are a relatively new arrangement where selected physicians and hospitals are recommended by employers or third parties to employees as preferred over other sources of medical care.  Any employee using these "preferred providers" receives more extensive health insurance coverage than the standard company plan.  The preferred providers typically agree to a fee schedule and some sort of utilization controls, and the hospitals agree to lower rates. In return, the providers receive payment more promptly and perhaps attract more patients or retain those who might be inclined to shift to an HMO or other less costly source of medical care.  The PPO differs from the HMO in that it does not lock in patients to receive their care from one set of providers; it does not guarantee availability of medical services; the providers are not necessarily assuming the financial risk; and there are no standard benefit packages.

PPO arrangements are increasing in number, particularly where HMOs are already a major competitive force, including Denver, Southern California, the San Francisco Bay area, and Texas.  They are of interest to health insurers because they promise survival in the face of HMO competition.  PPOs change the nature of the health insurance business since success will depend on who can identify and motivate the most cost-effective physicians and hospitals. In the past, competition in health insurance has been based on the ability of companies to rapidly process claims and to keep administrative costs down.  In my opinion, the PPO is a very important new development that many providers and consumers not participating in the HMO movement may find attractive.

As for HMO-like organizations, if the federal government broadens its definition of an HMO, I suspect the ultimate price competitive medical care organization may differ substantially from existing HMOs.  The most probable HMO-like organization that will develop is likely to provide rather comprehensive services, possibly even services beyond health care.  They will, however, resemble HMOs in the following manner:  (a) consumers will enroll for a specific period of time during which all their care is provided by the HMO, (b) the HMO will assume a position of risk as a fixed price contractor, and (c) the HMO will guarantee the availability of care.

I would further forecast that the health plans built around group practices are likely to dominate over the very large independent practice association (IPA) where physicians continue to operate in a solo practice fashion.  The latest InterStudy survey of hospital utilization by various types of HMOs suggests that large group practice plans are more successful than large IPAs in controlling hospitalization--the most costly facet of medical care. On the average, group practice plans experience 347 days, while the IPA plans experience 509 days of hospitilization per 1000.

Two kinds of adverse selection in large IPAs may influence their excessive hospitalization: adverse selection of patients and adverse selection of physicians. In the case of patients, IPAs tend to advertise the large number of participating physicians which means enrollees may not have to change physicians when they join. This advertising has the effect of attracting enrollees who have sought medical attention in the past and prefer a particular physician. This type of advertising may encourage a sicker population to join. In the case of adverse selection of physicians, the problem is not so much a qualitative problem as it is a quantitative one. The typical community of physicians does not necessarily match by specialty or numbers the needs of the population that joins the IPA. Facing an increasing supply of physicians, this poor match up between enrollee needs and physicians will make it increasingly difficult to control excess surgery, referrals and procedures.

Nonetheless, IPAs are an important element of the changing health care system. Faced with competiton from good group plans, physicians can quickly form an IPA and bring about widespread competition in a community. They are the only way HMOs can easily grow in communities where group practices are uncommon. However, I suspect that IPAs will either evolve into the preferred provider organizations previously described or will break up into smaller hospital-based units that more closely resemble group practices.

Perhaps the most important structural change in the health industry will be a shift in the delivery of physician services from local to nationally operated organizations. Already more than one half of the HMO services in the United States are delivered by national medical care organizations like Kaiser, INA, CNA and Prudential. If services provided by Blue Cross HMOs are added, then 64 percent of the HMO care is provided by larger organizations. This trend is likely to continue. However, the HMO business remains a difficult business, probably harder to manage than any other health enterprise. HMOs have very high capital requirements, especially in large cities; in fact, I think that explains why HMOs have not done as well as anticipated in cities like Philadelphia and Chicago. Because of these high capital requirements, large hospital medical groups and for-profit firms will likely dominate in this industry.

The presence of these national firms is important to the future of the health field. The more successful national firms will have a predictable performance record and will simply lay their template on city after city. National firms tend to have relatively high expectations—100,000 or more members. They will be attracted to the most wide open markets where no competition exists and where costs of medical care are already high. Prudential's PruCare pattern is illustrative; PruCare is in or entering Houston Dallas, Atlanta, Oklahoma City, Nashville, Tulsa and Chicago.

For competition to be effective, the competitive medical plans will have to involve at least 50 percent of the consumers in any given community; in fact, the Twin Cities' trends suggest that involvement might reach 60 to 75 percent. In the San Francisco Bay area, for example, participation has already reached 32 percent. Interestingly, that level of participation has not been sufficient to drive down the overall costs of medical care in the Bay area. However, systemwide effects by competitive medical plans may appear with enrollment as low as 20 percent. The key factor seems to be the proportion of practitioners involved in the plan, rather than the proportion of consumers involved.

Consider the impact of these new systems on the health industry, assuming that there are no major scientific breakthroughs that greatly alter the locale of medical care. Hospital utilization in the United States will drop to 750 days per 1000 over the next two decades, thereby reducing the number of beds required to about 2.5 beds per 1000 people. The need for physicians if these changes actually take place will be far less than the recent reports about the physician surplus predict. There will be a substantial change, too, in the distribution of health care dollars from 65 percent for hospital-related expenditures and 35 percent physician- related expenditures to the opposite distribution with physicians receiving approximately 65 percent of the health care dollar. The pattern of dollar distribution within HMOs in the Twin Cities has already changed; 35 percent or less of the health care dollar in each one of these plans goes for hospitalization and 65 percent to physicians.

The Pace Of Change

Even with radical shifts in public policy, health systems change extremely slowly. In Great Britain, people first began talking and writing papers about a national health service in 1911. It did not happen until 1948. Furthermore, Great Britain's health system changed following convulsive changes throughout the country—ravages of world war, a switch to socialism, and a collapse of the hospital system.

It appears to me that the most bullish competitive health system advocates have to recognize that two or more decades will be required for competitive market forces to dominate the American way of medical care. According to InterStudy's current projections, in ten years there will be 36 million people enrolled in competitive medical plans, and perhaps 150,000 physicians out of 600,000, providing care through these systems; at present 9.7 million people are enrolled and 50,000 physicians participate.

Consider how slowly the antecedents of this medical care revolution came into being. The Mayo Clinic, the forerunner of modern group practice, was built 75 years ago to provide tertiary care through a one-site delivery care system. The Kaiser Foundation Health Plan was established 40 years ago and continues to serve as a prototype for combining multispecialty and hospital care on a prepayment basis to provide comprehensive services. Kaiser brought scale to these changes as it was the first medical care organization in the United States to reach a billion dollar annual revenue.

The concept of competition as a national health policy and as a means of correcting market failure, has also been slow in evolving. The Federal Employees Benefit Program, which may be considered a prototype of fair market choice, is 20 years old. The Nixon health policy that advocated competition from a variety of delivery systems is ten years old. The emergence of any sort of a real competitive market, of which Minneapolis/St. Paul is an example, is five years old. Alain Enthoven's health plan is three years old. Preferred provider organizations are a year old. It must be recognized that these changes, although they start slowly in a community, acquire tremendous momentum because enrollment grows exponentially. The rate of enrollment that the Twin Cities is experiencing demonstrates how an exponential growth curve sneaks up on the inattentive observer. Although the enrollment in competitive medical plans has increased tenfold over the last ten years in the Twin Cities, competitive medical plans serve only 430,000 people. Now, however, the doubling time is approximately two and one-half years, and if current trends continue the number of people served will reach 800,000, or 40 percent of the market. In five years, 1.6 million people or 80 percent of the market will be served by competitive medical plans.

If we are to be guided by past experiences, the health industry is still evolving very slowly and it may take a long time before the American health system can be called "competitive." However, I would point out that once a medical marketplace heats up, so to speak, then very rapid changes take place and it is exceedingly difficult for organizations that have stayed out in the early stages to catch up. Certainly that has been the experience of the new medical care organizations in the Bay area that are attempting to compete with Kaiser.

## Forecaster's Clues

How can you, if you are sitting back and watching what is happening tell what is likely to happen? The following oddball clues are offered. First, the political clues. If President Reagan really does function like a chairman of the board, those chosen as health advisors will play an important role in shaping health policy. The Secretary of the Department of Health and Human Services makes far more difference to health matters than the President, and over the last ten years we have had several pro-competitive secretaries, namely Elliot Richardson and Joseph Califano. Secretary Schweiker previously introduced a pro-competitive bill in Congress. Another political clue has occurred in the Senate where there will be a change of membership and staffing of the health subcommittee of the Senate Finance Committee, now chaired by Senator Durenberger, a competition advocate.

A second important political change would be the passage of a capitation program for Medicare. Each Medicare enrollee in a competitive medical plan is equivalent in his impact on hospital demand to four to five employed individuals joining an HMO. The third important political clue would be the passage of a pro-competitive tax that capped health benefits. Perhaps a modification of the HMO Act could become simply a pro-competition health delivery reform act.

Second, private sector clues. The first major collective bargaining agreement between employers and employees accepting fair market choice will be significant. Under such an agreement, the contribution rate to all health plans would be equal and employees who choose a less costly alternative would receive either the savings or additional benefits. Imagine the significance of General Motors equalizing their contribution rate for employees so that employees who joined Kaiser at $110 a month would be allowed to keep the difference of $30-50 a month. Another private sector clue would be the overt promotion of health care competition by a leading corporation since industry tends to follow the leader.

In Memphis, conditions are right for a successful plan. Memphis is a large community whose hospital admission rates and utilization rates are double what a competitive medical plan would expect to experience. Memphis experiences 1754 hospital days per 1000; that figure can be lowered to 750. There is a very high per capita hospital expenditure, $409 per year, compared to the U.S. average in metropolitan areas of $344. Price competition will come when a major competitive health plan enrolls 25,000 people, grows at the rate of ten percent per year, and achieves a hospital utilization rate of 450 days or less per 1000. To be a real transforming force in the medical community, this competition must be capable of providing excellent medical care and preferably consist of highly respected physicians from the community.

Unfinished Business

First, what is the role of hospitals? No major competitive medical plan in the United States has been started and is still controlled by a hospital. It was probable that hospitals, as the major managers of capital and medical care in the health care industry, would enter this field, but they have not. My guess is that vertical integration of hospitals with medical groups is probably going to come into play very late in the process of health system reform and will be the result of competitive medical plans picking up hospitals rather than hospitals starting competitive medical plans. An exception to this statement is preferred provider organizations where much of the initiative is coming from hospitals.

Second, what is the role of academic medical centers? None of the successful HMOs in the United States could be called a main line business of an academic medical center, yet academic medical centers provide more than 25 percent of hospitalization to people over 65 in this country. How can an institution compete on price that is trying to cross-subsidize medical education and research from patient revenue? I am convinced they can compete if they try. The Mayo Clinic utilization data suggests they could compete on price now without changing anything except their mode of payment, but I know of no other academic medical center where integration of various specialties in the medical care system with education is sufficiently complete to compete with other well-run competitive medical plans.

So hospitals and academic medical centers remain large question marks for the future. I suspect that in both cases hospitals and medical education and research will come to competitive medical plans rather than those two types of medical institutions creating competitive medical plans.

Perhaps the most important need of the health system in the future is a genuinely contemporary model for medical care. The delivery arrangements currently being emulated are at least 40 years old. The key, I believe, is a commitment of this new segment of the health industry to research and development. Expenditures for health services research are only a hundredth of one percent in the United States. The health industry is not spending money to improve the quality of the product it delivers, and this revolution in medical care is not going to be very meaningful unless money is spent improving it. The momentum is there for an entirely new health care system. The real challenge for the 1980s is to create a better medical care system that produces excellent medical services.

What we need is a leader, a kind of medical care organization that succeeds because it provides the highest possible quality of medical care while giving people the sense that they are receiving personal service on a one-to-one basis.

# RESPONSE
## Carl J. Schramm

The task of following Paul Ellwood, who spews forth ideas like a volcano, is always difficult. Dr. Ellwood addressed three themes: conflict in the future of the health care delivery system, the problem of institutional change and the rate or pace of change. Looking at the question of conflict, it is critical that some of his forecasts be examined. It certainly bears repetition that the influence of the demands made by the health care system on society's total ability to produce is extraordinary. Ten years ago, the United States spent five percent of its gross national product on health care delivery and now spends ten percent. Some economic forecasts, produced by the Department of Health and Human Services, suggest that by 1990, 13 percent or more of the GNP will be spent on health care.

We know, as the opening days of the Reagan administration approach, that come Democrats or Republicans, the problem in the federal budget of an uncontrolled undiscretionary commitment to health care is a tremendous one. The solutions will be as hard to face for the incoming administration as they were for the outgoing administration. The projections which I assembled not too long ago with Bob Blendon from the Johnson Foundation are very sobering. In 1980, the federal government spent $80 billion on Medicare and Medicaid; roughly ten percent of the total federal budget. By 1985, the figure will be $110 billion or 13 percent of the budget. The historic trend of accelerated inflation rates in the health care delivery area is evidenced by the fact that the consumer price index (CPI) for medical care has exceeded the rate of increase in the CPI for all the goods and services in the economy for the last 30 years. This trend was interrupted in 1979 and 1980 by the pressures put on the economy by the cost of money, energy and housing and is predicted by economic forecasters to resume its 30 year trend by 1982.

I submit that these pressures spell conflict and the problems which will emerge will be severe. Conflict will be seen in the way institutions try to accomodate these pressures, and the federal government will face political problems in trying to merge interest groups which, as the 1980s unfold, seem to be unlikely collaborators. Hospitals, for example, have galloped forward with huge new construction projects, some underway and some already accomplished. These building projects require immense amounts of capital but this amount pales in light of the sums needed to operate the buildings after completion. Today as Dr. Ellwood pointed out, there is no basic research to indicate what the ratio of annual operating costs is relative to spending in terms of capital costs. This is a gross deficiency for policy-makers.

Providers clearly will have an ambiguous future. In 1970, 107 medical schools turned out 11,000 new physicians. By 1977, there were 134 medical schools turning out 18,000 new physicians. At the same time that we are attempting to shift the demand curve inward to dampen price inflation, we find ourselves with a new and much larger generation of physicians, most of whom have the same income expectations as the last generation. This alone will create immense conflict. One of the results of this conflict will be an increasingly ambivalent attitude toward the new allied health professions.

Obviously, taxpayers have a stake in all this and their concern seems to be evident when we consider the question of national health insurance. I suspect that if there is one anachronism that emerged from the presidential campaign year, it is the Kennedy-esque vision of a comprehensive national health insurance policy. Not only the members of the House of Representatives and the Senate, but also taxpaying citizens of the United States, stand in fear when they look at the huge financial expenditures needed for national health insurance relative to the experience of Medicare and Medicaid. They know this country cannot afford to support such a system. I think the conflict of the future will be severe and perhaps the gravest problem is that we lack ideas which have withstood the test of the market on any mass scale.

As to the second theme, institutional change, here I suspect the party most worthy of indictment is the American hospital. I think Dr. Ellwood is 100 percent right. We should have seen hospitals accomodate the notion of change in the marketplace. We should have seen hospitals, with their great power in the community, stepping forward with alternative plans of delivery and financing.

Institutional change is a terrible problem made more difficult because the hospital industry looks to be in better health than it was 15 years ago. Most hospitals are not in better health because of innovative structures adopted within hospital administration circles. Rather, they are financially healthier on the balance sheet, not withstanding the hoopla about failing hospitals in several northern inner cities, largely because the federal government has come aboard as a bride, paying anywhere between 40 and 50 percent of operating costs for many hospitals. Indeed, the only major change in the hospital system, and it is not one which hospital administrators can take credit for, is that in the last 15 years hospitals have reported profits. The decision to report these profits was made by trustees and administrators, not because it was important to make hospitals efficient, but because hospitals, to reach the private equity market for capital construction funds, had to appear as though they turned a profit. This is critical because hospital construction is inceasingly financed by public equity. Seven years ago, less than five percent of new hospital construction was built with public equity bonds, now over 55 percent of new construction is so funded. This is a radical change, and it is a change which spells great trouble in the future. We further tie the hospital to the general public economy, as Dr. Ellwood pointed out, by making pension funds increasingly dependent on the success and economic viability of hospitals. Another grave difficulty, as evidenced by New York City, is that in addition to producing health care, hospitals produce massive employment. This creates a political problem in shutting down unnecessary capacity.

The third theme is the rate of change. In the last 15 years, there has been great change in the health care industry. In addition to public equity support for hospitals, there has been a much greater change in what society expects of its hospitals. By and large, 15 years ago hospitals were conceived of as private, charitable institutions that had to be protected as special institutions in society. That attitude has changed. Hospitals are now regarded much like other corporations, and when analyzed in the light of the law, look like Ford, General Motors and Chrysler. Fifteen years ago, the charitable exemption for hospitals existed in many states; it is gone in most today. Fifteen years ago, the hospital judged its success and viability for the future by measuring whether or not it would have a balanced budget or a small enough deficit to be covered by its charitable endowment. That has changed. With the coming of Medicare and Medicaid as financing sources for operating revenues, hospitals instead of adjusting long-term goals toward just making it into the next year or two, began to build and to build big. Hospitals are no longer treated with special favor in collective bargaining, safety requirements and in public governance.

Before leaving the issue of institutional change, it should be noted that hospitals merit immense amounts of research in the years ahead; research that must be directed towards how the ownership interest, the interest of trustees, and community expectations of hospitals can be restructured so that at least 20 percent of current hospital bed capacity can be taken out of the system. If Dr. Ellwood is right, and I am inclined to believe he is, perhaps as much as 40 or 50 percent of current capacity needs to be eliminated.

Before closing, I want to make several comments about regulation. In certain states, partly because there are no models that seem able to spell short run relief, the notion of state regulation will flower. Limited recent studies indicate that in a small handful of states, regulatory attempts by the state legislature and the executive branch to control the rising cost of health care have been somewhat successful. The rates of inflation in six or seven northeastern states seem to be significantly lower in the light of three or four years of experience with hospital rate setting agencies. In the long run, however, I believe these agencies hold no hope. The only hope is to restructure the market. However, in the short run, it is probably inevitable that several more states adopt this approach. Indeed, a year or two after the beginning of the Reagan administration, there may be at least a tacit federal effort to stimulate the growth of these efforts in certain select states. The reason being, that state regulation may be a short run fix. Unfortunately, the short run fix may in the long run, create its own problems. For example, if ever there was a laboratory to look at the problems of regulation it is New York, where many of the problems resulting from five years of tightly constraining the rate of inflation are beginning to show acutely. One of the reasons these problems are acute is because no one has had the fortitude to speak clearly about the main issue in New York which is that there are at least 20 percent too many hospitals in the state. No one has spoken clearly to the citizenry about this problem because no one quite understands that the bullet has to be bitten right in half by a set of hard teeth.

Nevertheless, even knowing these things about regulation, some states will look to it as a solution. As they venture out into this area, certain things should be made clear to them about the nature of regulation. First, states are much different, one from the other; the south really is different from the northeast. Consequently, different regulatory approaches are needed. One of the problems is that the northeast seems almost intractable in its insistence to stick with the old model of care. There are big cities in the northeast which would be right for health maintenance organizations (HMO), yet in several of them, for example, Baltimore, the HMO concept does not seem to work very well. The entire power league of these communities seems wedded to large teaching institutions, the growth of small community hospitals of marginal quality, and the continued brinkmanship in the state budget process created by demands of the Medicaid entitlement program.

Second, state regulation may comport with the Reagan administration's emphasis on state solutions. Again and again it is said that one of the actions that will be taken is to give block grants to the states, thus placing more discretion in the hands of governors. Once that comes to pass, governors and not the President, will be faced with the hard choices of health policy, and one of the effective choices that has been made in a small number of states is the regulatory solution.

Third, as new hospitals are planned, a system which is neutral or even negative to the continued growth of the hospital system must be established. Most planning agencies are captives of the hospital system. The recent terrible experience in Baltimore of the planning agency disallowing outpatient surgical services throughout the entire central Maryland region is a scandal. Particularly when the reason for the disapproval is that existing hospitals have excess surgical capacity. I suggest that unneeded hospitals in major cities must be allowed to go bust. Mergers and other cosmetic attempts to bring poorly run and obsolete hospitals together

must be analyzed very carefully to determine if it would be better
for some of these hospitals to be closed.

Fourth, any regulatory system must insist on letting hospitals
make their own decisions with regard to management and the bottom
line.  Budget review, substituting state bureaucrats for hospital
administrators and trustees, is bound to fail, and will produce a
system more cumbersome, convoluted and difficult than that which
presently exists in a non-regulatory state.

Finally, the system that emerges in states which adopt a regulatory approach must be neutral as to payment sources.  That is to
say, these regulatory systems must at least allow, if not
stimulate, the development of pro-competitive plans such as HMOs
and independent practice associations.

In conclusion, these remarks may be viewed as piling bad news on
bad news, but there is some light in all of this.  Winston
Churchill wrote that in time of war allies will accomodate the
needs of each other which in peacetime they would find abhorrent.
I suggest that as we face a future filled with conflict over the
issues of regulation and competition, we really are on the brink
of war.  But being on the brink may bring accomodation, and this
is probably the bright light in the future.

# IX
# READINESS OF PUBLIC
# TO MANAGE OWN HEALTH CARE
## M.K. DuVal

Health education, what is it all about?  The professionals define
health education as any sequence of learning opportunities or experiences that, as a consequence of achieving a voluntary change
in behavior, culminates in better health.  The key is to recognize
that those matters pertinent to one's health come under one's personal control, and that one can make a judgment to change behavior
leading to better health.  The movement has roots back to 2000 BC.
For our purposes, the roots of the health education movement in the
United States surfaced late in the 19th century with well-baby clinics and health volunteers, and in the early 20th century with hygiene programs.

Hygiene's identity has been with athletics, physical education and
recreation for some time.  During the last 20 years there has been
a tremendous momentum of a new type in the health education movement.  It is this new type of health movement that will be discussed.

At the time of the White House Conference on Aging, the social aspiration that access to health care services ought to be a right
was adopted.  In the 1960s, those in a position to translate that
aspiration into public policy, found it a hard task.  They took two
steps.  First, they tried to eliminate money as a barrier to access
through the enactment of Medicare and Medicaid.  Second, they expanded the capacity side of the delivery system, so that no matter
what demand arose, it could be met.  New medical schools, public
health schools, osteopathic schools, dental schools and nursing
schools were built.  New investments in biomedical research were
made.  The National Institutes of Health budget went from $200
million to $2.2 billion in approximately 15 years.  Emergency
medical services and regional medical programs were developed.
Comprehensive health planning was promoted.  Community mental health
centers and neighborhood health centers were supported.  Everything
was tried in the 1960s.  It was a smorgasbord of opportunity, representing a staggering investment.  The result was that more

people received better medical care.  At the same time, the technological imperative and more scientific medicine were introduced.
Costs were driven up and the point of diminishing returns was
reached.  More and more money was being spent on individual cases,
without the purchaser seeing a return on that investment.

Even more serious, in my judgement, is that the profile of illness
and the causes of mortality changed.  Most of those ailments with
which we are currently afflicted as we go through life are, in many
instances, related to the choices we make in terms of how we are
going to live.  Will we smoke?  Will we exercise?  Will we follow
a diet resulting in obesity or being underweight?

As a consequence of the results that flowed from the transfusion
of the 1960s, where we grossly overdid it, we came into the 70s and
said, "Hold it, it didn't work, let's back up."  We began an era of
restraint, control and regulation.  As might be expected, the research investment was decreased; regional medical programs were
repealed; comprehensive health planning lapsed and was replaced
with health planning and development; support of health manpower
education was withdrawn; new health facility construction was halted;
and Professional Standards Review Organizations, certificate-of-
need, rate review, rate setting, hospital revenue caps and other
cost controls were introduced.

Fortunately, in addition to backing up, we did something else.
In 1971, the President questioned the role of the individual citizen
in addressing the issue of health care access as a right.  Why had
he or she not been a partner in the consideration of the evolution
of the translation of this aspiration into public policy?  As a result, the President established a Committee on Health Education,
and appointed Joe Wilson, the Chief Executive Officer at Xerox
Corporation, as Chairman.  The committee concluded first that it
was time people understood that health, in the last analysis, is
of value in its own right.  It is not enough to treat it passively
and when it is gone, call your physician.  Second, since so many
problems that relate to health are related to the way one chooses
to live, it is very important that people at least have a basis
of information from which to make informed judgments to maintain
good health.  The issue was not whether they made right or wrong
decisions, but that they made informed ones.

To do this, an entity called the National Center for Health Education was created in the private sector.  The Center is three years
old and has undertaken to see if it can fulfill that mission.

The movement toward health education that has captured our attention
has received tremendous momentum and support from many different
quarters including organizations such as the Academy of Pediatrics,
the American College of Physicians, the American Hospital Association, the American Medical Association, the National League for
Nursing and the American Dental Association.  These groups support
the Center financially, as well as supporting the health education
movement.  Voluntary health agencies are also pushing this movement.

Other interested parties are universities and colleges. They are starting to recognize that health education is, in fact, a discipline that requires research and standing within academia. Junior colleges, four year colleges and universities are beginning to give health education a standing in its own right by pulling it away from athletics. They are investing dollars in the new program, training people at the doctorate level, and doing research on the outcome of good health education and health promotion. Today there are over 250 approved programs in health education on campuses across the United States. There are even national associations of health educators, eight at last count.

Industry, upset over loss of productivity, poor worker morale, absenteeism and the increased cost of medical care benefits is looking hard at what it can do by showing an interest in employees and getting them to understand that health is their own concern and within their control. The list of large industries in the United States that have introduced extensive health programs for their employees is impressive and growing.

Government is also involved. The Bureau of Health Education has been created. The Office of Health Information and Health Promotion in the Office of the Assistant Secretary for Health coordinates all federal efforts in health education and health promotion. The Food and Drug Administration promotes patient package inserts to help consumers understand the effects of the drugs they are using.

The proprietaries are interested. Health education and promotion is a field in which money can be made. Addidas does not make shoes for altruistic reasons. Once the proprietary interest comes on board, it adds another force to the momentum of the movement.

I do not want to overlook the obvious, which is the interest at the level of the consumers. For convenience sake, they can be divided into two groups--the activist and the activated. The activist consumers are the Don Ardels and the Rick Carlsons and maybe extremists like Ivan Illich, whose book Medical Nemesis is a real waker-upper. These people are trying to say that one day we may be at a point where we realize that health and medical care are not the same. These activists have caught the public's attention. But more important are the activated consumers--the ones who are beginning to think about what they do, the way they live, and the habits they have chosen to adopt.

The movement is not without problems; it is neither a panacea nor the answer to every health problem.

First, health education does not yet rest on a scientific base. Using medicine as a parallel, there is simply no way to compare what is going on in health education. I cannot really tell you that changing your diet is going to lengthen your life. I cannot absolutely tell you that if you jog several miles a week you will live longer, happier, better or anything else. The point is that what we are doing at the moment is still selling a little bit of religion and a little bit of common sense. Until the scientific base catches up with the rhetoric, the movement has a problem.

Second, there are problems of territorialism and role delineation. Most physicians do not yet want any part of this in their offices, yet they fear that if they do not do it health educators will take over.  Nurses are involved in the same consideration.  Health educators cannot get along without the collateral strength that medicine can give, and yet they are frightened of being co-opted by medicine.  These territorial conflicts are real problems that could destroy the movement from the inside.

Third, there is the problem of the political and moral issues--the "do-gooding" phenomenon.  "You really ought not to smoke or drink. It is not good for you."  Whose value judgments should be accepted in these matters?  Many have an instinct to rebel against taking someone else's advice.

Fourth, the movement can lead to something that is a little dangerous--victim blaming.  Should the person who smokes pay a higher premium on his insurance?  Should the person who is more than ten percent overweight be taxed?  The issue of victim blaming assumes that a person can control his own destiny and all of his habits.

Thus there are important moral issues about the choices one makes in terms of living, and whether or not one should be a free agent in making a decision to do, or not to do, something.  They involve the imposition of someone else's value judgments, and the ultimate issue of what is in the public interest when contrasted with the private right to be free to make one's own life decisions, a basic American question.

The ultimate question would be at what point can the spending of tax dollars to change someone's behavior be justified?  The book A Clockwork Orange is one of the most dramatic presentations of the thesis that there may come a point at which behavior can become so reprehensible that it justifies the intrusion of the state in controlling that behavior.

A fifth problem is funding.  Nobody wants to pay for it.  Health is not a sickness benefit; it is not an insurable event.

Finally, and perhaps most importantly, is that leading a self-conscious healthy life is afoul of the culture we live in.  Our contemporary culture is inimical to good health.

I was fascinated not long ago while watching the Academy Awards that the one common theme of every motion picture honored was stress, exactly what health education works to get rid of.  I am fascinated by the fact that, today, one of the hotter items of concern is junk food, and the cocktail hour is still part of the normal day.  Also, the degree to which violence and pornography are acceptable cannot be good for a person's mental health.

Furthermore, we have a television oriented society.  Recent figures indicate that by the time a child is through high school he has had 15,000 organized hours of instruction and over 18,000 hours of exposure to television.  This includes as many as 300,000 television commercials.  The point of many of these commercials is that you do not have to solve any of your own problems, just go down to the store and get a box of X. Over a period of time the effect of these commercials and the dependency they may breed becomes great.

Thus, the important questions are: Is the public ready to manage its own health? Is it ready to assume an intelligent and sophisticated posture in choosing between competing offerings? Is it ready to become an informed collaborator?

I conclude that we have a long way to go. On the other hand, I think the public is substantially ahead of where most professionals think it is, and that we professionals must catch up to it.

# X
# RACONTEUR
## John A. Shively

It is difficult to summarize in ten minutes the tremendous program that has been presented during the past three days. Therefore, I will touch on some of the highlights and then Dr. Enthoven will discuss the areas that would best be addressed in some detail.

Senator Durenberger opened the Forum with a superb presentation on the politics of health. He pointed out that there are no partison politics in health care, and that health care politics can be managed by competition and consumer choice. He further noted that new and better ways to deliver public services, including health care, are needed. The government's role should be as a policy-maker with users making the choice among programs in a competitive health care delivery system.

He also pointed out something I had not previously appreciated, that we are in the midst of a cycle to decrease the role of government in delivering services with change dependent on "voice" and "exit." The "exit" choices need to control inflation and stabilize income. These, of course, are allied needs that are identified in the graying population of retirees in this country.

During the ensuing discussion, the question was raised about the Durenberger bill, which has a monetary limit of tax credit rather than level or unit of medical care in order to provide equity in different geographic areas of the United States due to differences in fees and costs. This question was later identified for discussion in some of the workshop sessions.

Dr. Farmer in the opening comments the following day made the succinct statement that the choices were really only two--regulation with constraints or regulation with competition. He also identified problems of academic health science centers with regulations, and expressed concern regarding the primary mission of the centers. He almost had a posture of a suppliant asking, "Oh Lord, who's responsibility is it to take care of indigent patients? When and where were academic health science centers charged by society with this responsibility?"

Subsequently, Dr. Enthoven gave the theme address on competition in the marketplace.  First he reviewed health care cost increase factors, as well as the ineffectiveness of the methods used by cost containment, certificate-of-need, PSRO, and physician/fee control. He proposed several treatments for cutting costs without decreasing quality of care:  (1) matching resources to needs, (2) appropriate regionalization of specialized services, (3) decreasing hospitalization utilization per capita, (4) decreasing the length of stay in hospitals, (5) simple cost consciousness, and (6) enlisting the physician in devising cost conscious systems.  The principles of competitive systems were enumerated such as multiple choices and fixed dollar subsidies with adjustment for inflation, rules applied equally and competitors and physicians organized in competing economic units.  The change in the health care system must be in incremental steps rather than through a complete revision of the present system by Congress.  He also noted that "tinkering" with the health care system generally has no appreciable effect on cost.

Robert Derzon pointed out that the higher the cost of health care, the greater the support of the aged and poor by the government, and the greater the regulatory constraints by the same. He pointed out again that the physician is in a pivotal position in controlling the cost of care.  He critiqued Enthoven's plan, noting that (1) the poor, aged and sick are left out of the plan, (2) competition is not easily developed in the health care field, especially in an area of a monopoly, (3) competition may not bring down prices, and (4) industry and labor are often not willing to change their collective bargaining position.  He reviewed the impact of competition on medical schools and health science centers, including the loss of insurable patients who go elsewhere, the tertiary service emphasis, educational cost identification, and the increased efficiency of care and education that needs to be present in university hospitals as well as community hospitals gradually withdrawing from graduate medical education which is concentrating in academic health centers.

There were a series of papers on health plan groups which Dr. Enthoven will discuss.  I might, however, make several general comments.  First, the presentation by Mr. Johnston described a unique plan for pooling funds from multiple sources that results in contracts with providers for complete health services to the poor. This plan acts as a broker, with consumer choice of plan.  In response, Mr. Turner pointed out that in Memphis the indigent lack a competitive alternative and there is a general lack of acceptance of the voucher system for health care because of the hazard of extending this system to private primary and secondary schools.

Second, Dr. Simmons predicted that competition would occur regardless of the Enthoven plan because both industry and unions are convinced that the cost of health care is too high as well as much being neither beneficial or effective.  Third, Dr. Ellwood discussed the American way of medical care for the 1980s, and Dr. Schramm responded by pointing out that at the current rate of change, there would be a goal of a 20 to 40 percent decrease in hospital beds within the next decade or two.  And finally, Dr. DuVal reviewed the problems with health education and prevention.

The work sessions were composed of delegates representing a wide variety of backgrounds for input into the discussion of forces moving and also impeding competition. This very background also brought up some specific areas of concern: What will it do to me, and perhaps what is in it for me and the group that I represent? I think it represents the basic fact that when you have individuals with experience, you also have prejudices and biases.

It would be difficult to summarize or identify the essence of the small group discussions. If there was one thing that was gratifying to see in several group discussions, it was the conclusion that we cannot afford not to move ahead!

I would like to end by focusing on Dr. McClure's address on national health policy for the 1980s. He focused on the precise connotation of market reform versus economic regulation pointing out that with increased market forces there is inevitable decrease in regulation and with decreased market forces there is increased regulation by the public utility route. He noted that if we have the option, we should avoid the posture of supporting competition but really meaning status quo. This is really not an option, since the 1980s will bring about change. He also raised the question of what does fair market and effective competition really mean? I am reminded of the need, during the past decade, for medical and health educators to acquire educational methodology as well as to understand what is meant by much of the jargon used so freely. I predict that in the next decade, medical educators need to conquer medical economics and marketing so that they understand the subtleties of what is meant by fair market, effective competition, marginal costs and opportunity costs.

Some general overall perceptions can be identified as to the future. We need a combination of competition and regulation with a proper balance and effective links. The objective or challenge is that expressed by Charles Schultz and quoted by Dr. Enthoven, "the public use of private interest." I think we will have to accept that there has to be management of the conflicting forces of competition and community needs, that regulation is used as a force to keep the market honest, and that the either or syndrome should be replaced with the and also concept.

# XI
# CLOSURE
# Alain C. Enthoven

I will review a few thoughts I have collected based on what I have heard in interacting with the various workshop groups and in other discussions with Forum participants. First, I have heard concern over how these ideas of delivery system reform through competition relate to the indigent, that is to say Medicaid beneficiaries and other poor people, and I have several points to make about that. One, everyone must recognize that the fiscal squeeze on government is real and is worsening. Senator Durenberger spoke about Proposition 13 and the taxpayers' revolt. This is a real problem and is exemplified by the simple fact that graduates of the Stanford Business School, young men and women in their late twenties, leave the campus and step off into the 50 percent marginal tax bracket. That used to be something thought of as a privilege for rich people, and now young professionals are starting out in that position. It is intolerable. It means that they have no hope of saving enough money to make a down payment on a house. It is something that is not going to endure.

Real corporate retained earnings in this country in the past decade have been incredibly low. The tax system does not make corrections for the impact of inflation on inadequate depreciation allowances. As a result, there is a crisis of lack of investment because of lack of profitability with the result of an absolute decline in productivity. This is a very ominous trend that simply must be reversed. Savings and productive investment in the economy are by far the lowest of the industrialized nations. Americans once prided themselves on America's superior economic growth. Now the country is falling behind, and I think it is because of the heavy tax burden on industry and the disincentives for saving that Senator Durenberger discussed.

You may say, "I have heard about this before. We have been talking about health care costs at least since I was a kid--so what is new now?" What is new is the sheer size of the outlays for health. Medicare doubling was no big deal when Medicare cost $1 or $2 billion a year or $9 billion per year in 1972. But at today's $35 billion per year cost, the next doubling is going to be a big deal,

even though a billion dollars does not buy what it used to. I think
the well is dry; there is no more blood in the turnip. The attitude
of the 1960s--oh well, we can just raise the taxes--is gone, as indicated by the election returns.

My second comment regarding care of the indigent is that the present
delivery system presents a paradox of excess and deprivation. So
often medical residents have said to me: "We have a Medicaid patient in the hospital. I would not let them do to my own mother
what they did to him. They did three CAT scans, including a con-
trast-enhanced scan, etc." Once they are covered, these patients
receive a whole lot of high technology medicine, much of which is
not efficacious or necessary. At the same time, people who are
not covered often lack access even to basic, urgently necessary
primary care. Thus there is this paradox of excess and deprivation.

I think there are two ways to respond to the fiscal squeeze. One is
to keep the present system and see the budget balanced by cutting
eligibility and benefits. I think this would be a tragedy, but it is
going to happen. At least in California it will occur since the state
already has constitutional limits on spending and balanced budget
requirements. Medicaid in California will probably hit $5 billion
next year, and the state will run out of money for the program. One
way or another it will be shut down.

The alternative that is still possible to adopt, is simply to cut the
waste and build a cost-effective system for all people. We can
afford to care for the poor if the care for everyone is economical.
My vision is that all the poor would be given a subsidized choice of
competing HMOs and other similar alternative delivery systems that
serve the general population. This would be mainstream care which
would solve the problem of access. HMOs' strong point is often
access, that is why so many people join them. They know any time,
day or night, if they need a physician, there will be one within
instant reach. Diana Dutton, my Stanford colleague, has done studies
of access to care for low income, inner-city families in Washington,
D.C. and found that the patients who belong to HMOs have the best
access.

There is some experience to show ways this can be done. For example,
I read Mr. Johnston's experience in Multnomah County, Oregon as
being promising. In California, there is some contracting with HMOs
and it does definitely save the state money; money which can be used
to extend benefits to more people. There are problems that have to
be solved, especially the problem of cycling in and out of eligibility as income fluctuates, and the accompanying adverse risk
selection. There must be a way to stabilize membership in an HMO for
at least a year if the government wants it to work. Where eligibility is steady, no serious cycling problem exists. I am not pro-
posing or asking for a cross-subsidy. If an HMO is asked to
accomodate a higer-risk group, it can be done through an adjusted
community rate. For example, if an HMO enrolls an aged, blind and
disabled group whose predicted utilization is twice that of other
enrollees, the HMO should be allowed to charge twice its market
tested ordinary community rate.

I believe the only way to make mainstream care affordable for the poor is to make it cost-effective for all of us. There is nothing anti-poor in this concept. On the contrary, I think it is their last best hope.

The next general point I would like to address is the question: Is this all real or is it theory? A frequent reaction that I have heard here and elsewhere is: "That is an interesting theory, but I wonder what it would be like if we tried all those ideas. Will they work?" In one of the workshop groups, I heard a very logical rational explanation that leads to the conclusion they cannot work. It is sort of like an aeronautical engineer who gives an analysis and ends up with the statement: "The bee can't fly." Other people say, "These are very interesting ideas. Try a demonstration somewhere, but not here." What the speakers at this Forum have said is that bees now fly in California, in Minnesota, in Hawaii, in Oregon and in other areas of the country. There have been large scale long-term demonstrations with these ideas. HMOs are not an experiment; they are here to stay. They are established successful enterprises that do the job for considerably less cost. This is not something weird or second-rate; it is commonsense and first-rate.

HMOs do very well with educated middle-class consumers. They have very high market shares in places like Control Data Corporation, and the faculties of Stanford University and the University of California. I think the reason that HMOs do very well with this educated middle and upper income segment is because these people recognize that good quality and economy usually go hand in hand. In the case of hospital utilization, for example, we have noted that both the Mayo Clinic and Kaiser Permanente Medical Care Program hospitalize their people some 40 percent <u>less</u> than the national average. I believe as far as quality of good care is concerned that the Kaiser-Mayo standard is the gold standard. If you look at how these organizations save money, it is through regional concentration of specialized services, outpatient surgery, unit medical records, and matching the number of surgeons to the needs of the population served, which means proficient surgeons. All these actions improve the quality, and incidentally cut the cost, of care.

Finally, on this theme, competition does work. Where people have choices, they do consider price as well as other variables. HMO market shares do grow well where there is a fair choice. The problem is most people do not have a fair choice.

My next main point is that the competitive strategy is a way of helping cost-effective organized systems of care grow by letting the people who form and join them get the savings--something absent in the dominant insured fee-for-service system. It is a way of harnessing self-interest. It is the invisible hand described by Adam Smith. A reward to people for making economical choices--they get the savings. Competition is a strategy and some principles which have to be adapted to local circumstances. It is not a rigid orthodoxy or a magic formula.

In conclusion, it seems that it is time now for the professionals in Memphis to act. The large employers ought to sit down with representatives from Health First and from Blue Cross/Blue Shield's Memphis Health Care Corporation so that these plans can be offered to employees on the same basis as the employer's current plans are offered.  Of course, employers must first review the quality and financial solvency of the plans and resolve all questions any prudent buyer would normally raise.  If the answers to these questions are not positive, then employers need to work with the plans to resolve the problems.  After the plans are acceptable, everyone must work to protect them.  That is, keep them from being blocked by boycotts or by non-cooperation.  For example, a couple of years ago I visited with the Harvard University Community Health Plan staff.  One of its biggest difficulties was that at a number of the hospitals in the community, the medical staffs would vote unanimously to deny hospital privileges to any physician participating in Harvard's Plan.  And of all the incredible hypocrisy, they said it was on the grounds of quality.  Now these physicians all have faculty appointments at Harvard so there must have been something more to the denial.

I know this goes on in every community.  Hospitals say they would like to work with the HMOs but their medical staffs threaten to take their patients to another hospital if they do.  Civic leaders must be alert to this and recognize it as wrong.  It is not the American way.  Hospitals should be able to deal with the HMOs on the grounds of rational mutual advantage.

The time to act is now.  The longer a community waits, the harder it will be to solve the problems, and they will not go away by themselves.

I hope that in two or three years there will be another Norfleet Forum on "Competition in the Health Marketplace" and that I will have the pleasure of coming to Memphis to learn about the successful launching of several new, cost-effective organized systems of care.

# APPENDIX A:
## Trustees, Director, and University Officials

For The University of Tennessee
Center for the Health Sciences:

Bland W. Cannon, M.D.
Special Advisor to the Chancellor

James C. Hunt, M.D.
Dean, College of Medicine

Stephen T. Miller, M.D.
Associate Professor of Community Medicine
College of Medicine


For the Memphis-Plough Community Foundation:

George M. Houston
Chairman of the Board
Mid-South Title Insurance Company
Memphis, Tennessee

Edward W. Reed, M.D.
General Surgery
Memphis, Tennessee


Forum Director:

James R. Gay, M.D.
Associate Vice President for Health Affairs
The University of Tennessee


Officers of the University:

Edward J. Boling, Ph.D.
President
The University of Tennessee

T. Albert Farmer, Jr., M.D.
UTCHS Chancellor
Vice President for Health Affairs